ARM CARE

A Complete Guide To Prevention and Treatment of Tennis Elbow

D1178536

Robert P. Nirschl, M.D., M.S.
Janet Sobel, P.T.

Published by
Medical Sports, Inc.
Publications Division
P.O. Box 7187
Arlington, VA 22207

NOTE: The information contained in this book is not intended to be prescriptive. Any attempt to diagnose, treat, or rehabilitate an injury or disorder should come under the direction of a physician or orthopedic specialist.

ISBN: 0-912261-04-8

Library of Congress Catalog Card No. 93-081184

Dedication

To All Patients . . .

. . . who in life and athletics (whether performing arts, occupational, or sports) have succumbed to, or will be prevented from succumbing to the maladies described in this book.

Contents

Acknowledgements

Much of medicine is a labor of love. This book is no exception. For us to share what we have learned takes committment and sacrifice by many others among my staff and family. Some do not necessarily share our same enthusiasm for the project but selflessly carry on and contribute anyway.

Janet Sobel and the professional Physical Therapy Staff at Virginia Sports-medicine Institute have been a constant source of improved knowledge [base] and protocol refinement. The efforts of Ellen Maquire, Lisa Phillips and Diane Cooney concerning this project are especially noteworthy. The secretarial support and word processing skills of Jacci Duncan is very much appreciated. Nancy Howard has contributed significantly in her graphic skills. Suzanne Nirschl Brown has added significantly wonderful insight. Donna Benson-Chan and Dawn Curry deserve special kudos for bringing the technical aspects of the project to fruition.

Finally, a special thanks to my wife, Mary Ann, and the rest of the family who have accepted the familiar pose of Dad at the beach, in our home library, or wherever, with pen and pad in hand.

Preface

As with all areas of medicine, the world of tendon injuries has undergone major transition. Since our first book, *Arm Care,* was published in 1981 conceptual knowledge of these injuries has increased dramatically. In addition, the practical implementation and sophistication of the Nirschl Orthopedic/Sportsmedicine Clinic and the Virginia Sportsmedicine Institute diagnosis and rehabilitation programs have been markedly improved.

The refinement in our understanding of the basic anatomy and phases of pathological change, as defined by degree of tissue abnormality, has been particularly helpful. This understanding now allows us the luxury of more accurately forcasting the expected outcome of a particular treatment for an individual patient. The distinction and recognition of "failed healing patterns" now allows us to define the surgical candidate earlier thereby eliminating prolonged and likely unproductive rehabilitation efforts.

The constant goal of any quality tendinitis treatment should be to identify abnormal (pathological) tissue and amend this tissue in a positive manner, while enhancing, or at least protecting, adjacent normal tissue. In reviewing many rehabilitation programs, including both orthodox physical therapy and unorthodox approaches, it has been amazing to us how often these concepts are not recognized resulting in a protocol which is nothing more than an uncoordinated trial and error approach.

This book recounts our experience at the Nirschl Orthopedic/Sportsmedicine Clinic and Virginia Sportsmedicine Institute in treating literally thousands of tennis elbow tendinitis patients. We have learned which treatments offer the best opportunities for success, which do not, and how long rehabilitation should take. We have also learned that since the location and magnitude of pathological change varies greatly, utilizing "one cook book approach" is likely to yield inconsistent results. It is critical to understand, therefore, that there is "no substitute for individualization."

The principles in this book are applicable to the treatment of other areas of tendinitis/tendinosis, and we have accumulated substantial experience in other anatomical locations including the shoulder, knee, shin, ankle and foot. This wealth of rehabilitation information will receive attention in future publications. You will note that the term tendinosis has been introduced alongside the common term tendinitis. We now know that microscopic examination of injured tissue fails to identify an inflammatory process, thus the term tendinitis is a misnomer. This fact, in addition to many other concepts introduced in this book, may come as a surprise even to competent medical professionals. This should not be surprising, as medical information, by its nature, progresses rapidly. It is our hope that you will benefit greatly from what we have learned thus far.

Chapter I

Tennis Elbow
Definition and Causation

"Tennis elbow" seems to make its first appearance in the English literature in the 1880's. The term, however, has been much maligned over the intervening century. When we initiated research into this problem in 1967, we were surprised to discover that several medical articles stated that the malady rarely occurs in tennis players. Finding medical statements of such inaccuracy was a powerful stimulus to get the facts straight concerning this curious yet highly distressful malady.

It should be noted that in many instances tennis elbow is not an isolated malady. Indeed, many associated problems either result from, or result in, tennis elbow. For example, shoulder injury may ultimately result in elbow injury or vice versa. Commonly associated problems include:

1. shoulder tendinitis/tendinosis,
2. neck arthritis,
3. ulnar nerve pinch at the elbow,
4. median nerve pinch at the wrist, known as carpal tunnel syndrome,
5. wrist overload (triangular fibrocartilage complex and distal radial-ulnar joint overload),
6. multiple areas of tendinitis/tendinosis (such as both shoulders and elbows) known as "mesenchymal syndrome" and
7. injury and strength deficiencies in the legs, back and shoulder.

Although this book is specifically directed to the prevention and treatment of tennis elbow, it is critical to understand when other maladies, such as those listed above, are present, these problems must be addressed with targeted treatment and exercise programs in association with the tennis elbow program.

Medical considerations

The medical description and the anatomy of tennis elbow are divided into three areas: lateral, medial and posterior. Lateral is the most common, followed by medial (the ratio of lateral to medial is approximately five to one) and posterior, which is relatively uncommon (except in baseball pitchers and serious weight lifters).

The usual tennis elbow is a painful alteration of tendons referred to as tendinitis, or, more appropriately, tendinosis. Lateral tennis elbow is extensor tendinosis (primarily extensor carpi radialis brevis). Medial tennis elbow is flexor tendinosis (primarily flexor carpi radialis and pronator teres). Posterior tennis elbow is triceps tendinosis (often associated with posterior elbow chondromalacia arthritis.) See illustrations, pg. 3.

The spectrum of tendinosis may vary widely, from slight inflammatory irritation to a full blown major change in the entire tendon, including rupture. This explains why one person will respond quickly to a case of tennis elbow and others respond slowly, or not at all, without surgery. Determining the magnitude of pathological tendon change often requires the expertise of a physician who has extensive experience in treating tendon injuries. Modern laboratory aids which image soft tissues, such as ultrasonography and MRI, may help in distinguishing the various stages of tendinosis. The use of these techniques are still in the investigational stage, however.

There are levels of tendinitis/tendinosis, and determining the level of injury accurately will result in the prescription of the optimal treatment for a particular patient.

Levels of Tennis Elbow Tendinitis/Tendinosis
Nirschl System

Level	Evident Damage
I	Pain and/or chemical inflammation No permanent tendon change
II	Permanent tendon change - less than 50% tissue injury evident in tendon cross section
III	Permanent tendon change - greater than 50% tissue injury evident in tendon cross section
IV	Complete rupture of tendon

Symptoms of injury

Pain and tenderness, the major symptoms of tennis elbow, generally manifest themselves gradually. Tennis elbow symptoms occur most commonly among individuals between 35 and 50 years of age, for both males and females. Heavy forearm use, such as playing tennis 3-4 times per week, or occupational activities such as meat cutting or typing is common among tennis elbow sufferers. Pain associated with handshaking or simple activities such as picking up a cup are also common symptoms.

Location of the symptoms for the varieties of tennis elbow usually follow the outline indicated in the illustrations as demonstrated by X and arrow:

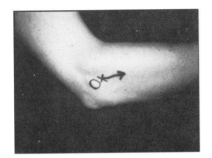

Lateral Tennis Elbow

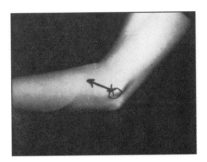

Medial Tennis Elbow

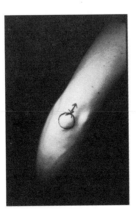

Posterior Tennis Elbow

Predisposing factors for injury - Who gets it?

Two categories of factors contribute to an individual's vulnerability to injury.

Category I
Physiological and Anatomical Factors: These factors are not easily altered.

A. Hereditarial body design (such as angles of muscle and tendons; e.g., exaggerated varus-valgus).
B. Associated body deficiencies arising from prior injury, disease, or other factors (such as strength deficiencies, gout and probably low estrogen levels in women). In addition, there is a small group of persons who appears predisposed to generalized tendinitis/tendinosis in various body parts. Symptoms are often present in both elbows, the shoulders and hands, commonly in association with nerve pinch problems at the elbow and wrist. This malady is known as mesenchymal syndrome and probably represents a subtle hereditarial alteration of tendon protein.
C. Age - the group from 35-50 years of age is most at risk.

Category II
Non-anatomical Factors: These factors usually are more easily altered.

A. Improper conditioning for a sport or activity:
　　Unfortunately, many recreational athletes invite injury by "taking up a sport to get in shape" rather than "getting in shape to take up a sport." Competitive athletes also make a serious mistake when they believe "playing their sport" is all that is required to maintain conditioning for a highly competitive level of activity.
　　The above mistakes are laden with injury producing danger. Adequately balanced forearm muscle strength, flexibility and endurance is essential. Equally important is the role of overall body function. The body operates as a linked system, getting energy from ground reaction and other physical forces and transferring it up through the legs, hips, and trunk to the arms. Although the elbow is often the area that suffers in racquet and throwing sports, injury here can often be attributable to deficits elsewhere. Both inadequate agility and a lack of balanced muscle strength in the legs and/or trunk can result in getting to the ball late which can result in tendinitis/tendinosis of the shoulder, elbow and wrist.

   B. Abusive overload (overuse):
1. Excessive intensity, duration or frequency of sport or occupational activity (playing or working too often, too long, or at too intense a level).
2. Sudden increase or change in intensity, duration or frequency.
3. Faulty sports or occupational techniques.
4. Inadequate warm-up and cool-down.
5. Poor equipment choices for the sport or occupational work place.

Faulty Techniques

As noted, activities which require heavy muscle work can result in abusive overload. The technique of muscle use plays an important role in health or injury. Every activity has a biomechanically proper technique, as well as, a slew of improper ones. In movements such as lifting or shaking hands, for example, occurrence of pain quickly informs the sufferer that there must be a better way. He or she will generally be able to change to a more comfortable technique; therefore, common sense modification of many daily activities is good medicine.

In contrast to abusive overload, regular, controlled and systematic arm use is necessary for good health and as a preventive measure against damage, and is an important aid in recovery from injury. In sports or occupational activities, a change of technique may often relieve symptoms and improve performance simultaneously.

Like the shoulder, the elbow is subject to multiple overload abuses secondary to technique inadequacies. The major error is using the smaller, less powerful forearm muscles for a job best done by the more powerful shoulder and trunk-leg muscles. This error has a high injury potential in sports and results in poor sports performance. Many recreational and occupational activities including tennis, golf, baseball, volleyball, track & field events, gardening, typing/computers, carpentry, repetitive lifting, performing arts and repetitive handshaking can be implicated in tennis elbow.

Techniques of Forearm Use

Lateral Elbow Overload

In the common lateral tennis elbow, the overload occurs in the forearm extensors (muscles on the back of the forearm which raise the wrist). One special muscle (the extensor brevis) seems to be affected most often because of its position and function. In tennis, this overload most commonly occurs during an incorrect backhand, but the serve and forehand can cause problems as well. The key point in the tennis backhand is to keep the elbow firm and *almost* fully extended (a small amount of elbow bend aids in shock absorption). Motion and power, therefore, come primarily from body weight transfer, trunk rotation and shoulder motion. The forearm muscles are used primarily for racquet control in a quality stroke.

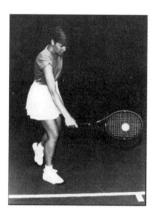

Quality Backhand

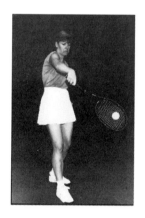

Faulty Backhand

Many other activities can result in lateral elbow overload. Careful assessment of these activities including sports, occupational, and performing arts with appropriate correction are pertinent to prevention and treatment.

Medial Elbow Overload

Medial tennis elbow overload occurs at the origin of the forearm flexors at the medial elbow, especially the pronator and the wrist flexors. Techniques which constantly require wrist snap and forearm pronation (e.g., a palm down twist as in a late forehand stroke in tennis, squash, volleyball spike, golf, baseball throwing, or the pull-through in swimming) are prime sports causes. Techniques which stretch the medial elbow (baseball pitching, a quality tennis serve or javelin throwing) are also major causes of medial overload.

Racquetball and squash techniques are usually forearm dominant (e.g., wristy strokes). Some protection is offered by the smaller ball and racquet, as compared to tennis. The techniques of these sports are definitely injury producing if applied to tennis.

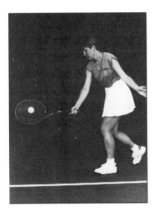

Quality Forehand

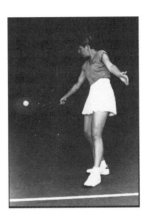

Faulty Forehand

Posterior Tennis Elbow

Posterior tennis elbow (triceps tendinitis/tendinosis) occurs with heavy and sudden elbow extension or straightening (usually a snapping motion such as the tennis serve, baseball pitching or weight lifting). The basic techniques may be correct, but a smoother and less snapping end point in the motion is needed. The bicep muscle may be weak, thereby not being able to smoothly control elbow extension resulting in a snapping elbow extension.

Throwing Motions

The pitching motion of adults and children is similar. Medial elbow overload in children can result in growth line disturbance commonly known as 'little leaguer's elbow," rather than tendinitis.

Some biomechanical techniques, as noted, are poor for both sports efficiency and arm health. Correction, therefore, results in improved sports ability, as well as, arm health. There are other movements, however, that may be quite effective as sports techniques, but still cause arm injury. These motions are harder to correct while maintaining the desired level of sports effectiveness. For the highly competitive athlete, this situation often requires quality coaching help, including slow motion video and possibly computer biomechanical analysis.

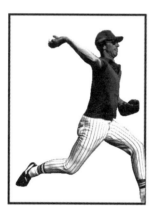

Punishing Motion

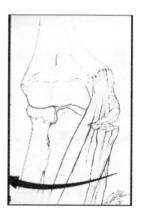

Effects of punishing motion:
Damage to medial tendons and ligaments

Little League Elbow

Much has been said about "little leaguer's elbow." This malady may be defined as an overuse irritation of the medial elbow growth line in children. The mechanism of injury is the same as with adult throwing, namely a stretching (valgus stress) of the medial elbow structures with throwing. In youngsters, the "open" growth line is more vulnerable than the tendon and ligament attachments.

The symptoms are similar to adult medial tennis elbow. X-rays usually show nothing, but can show minor to major changes of the medial growth line, and on occasion, lateral elbow compartment compression changes may also occur (osteochondritis dissecans).

Some past studies have suggested an incidence of "little leaguer's elbow" as high as 70% among little league pitchers. Recent studies including our own study indicate a very low incidence (4%).

Curve ball throwing has been anecdotally implicated as a technique cause of "little leaguer's elbow." The curve is imparted by variations in forearm twisting or rotation. In our studies, however, forearm rotation plays little role in medial elbow overload, leading us to conclude that curve ball throwing technique does not in itself cause injury).

The major causes of *little leaguer's elbow* are similar to *adult medial tennis elbow:*

1. Excessive throwing.
2. Horizontal arm elevation in the throwing technique.
3. Sharp wrist snap and forearm pronation (e.g., fast ball technique).
4. Elbow beyond 90° of extension at ball release (valgus angle).

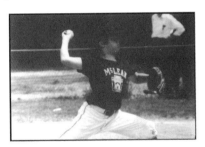

Punishing horizontal arm position

The treatment for "little leaguer's elbow" is similar to tennis elbow. In most instances, good results will occur with less throwing and better arm elevation in the throwing technique in association with rehabilitative exercise.

Golf Elbow

Golf, like the racquet, throwing, and swimming sports has a high incidence of shoulder and elbow problems. Lateral tennis elbow is especially common in the leading arm and medial tennis elbow in the trailing arm. Lateral elbow symptoms are magnified by the taking of excessive divots or slicing with iron shots. Medial elbow symptoms are intensified by an overly dominant trailing arm which often results in the ball being hooked. Wristy, rather than firm wrist techniques, are also punishing to the elbow tendons.

As in the other cited sports, total arm weakness and shoulder abnormalities in the forms of shoulder tendinitis, subluxation, and A-C arthritis are commonly associated with elbow abnormalities. To be totally effective, therefore, the rehabilitation efforts must encompass the entire arm, shoulder and upper trunk. A critical review of golf technique is also important to overall treatment success.

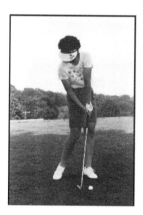

Golf stroke at ball impact. Lead arm is subject to lateral tennis elbow.
Trailing arm is subject to medial tennis elbow.

Highlights of Chapter 1

1. Tennis elbow is a painful tendinitis/tendinosis affecting specific tendons in specific areas of the elbow.
2. Three types of tennis elbow occur: lateral, medial and posterior. Lateral tennis elbow is the most common.
3. Common predisposing factors include:
   a. Age (35-50 years is most prevalent)
   b. Repetitive overuse of the dominant arm (playing tennis 3-4 times per week, occupations such as meat cutting, carpentry and typing or performing arts are examples)
   c. Sudden change in activity level (e.g. increased activities)
   d. Weakness of the relatively small forearm muscles associated with sport or occupational techniques which overload these small, weak muscles.
   e. Systemic hereditarial factors such as tendency to gout, low estrogen levels in females, and an unexplained predisposition to tendinitis/tendinosis (mesenchymal syndrome)

Chapter II

Pain

Without pain, minor injuries might quickly grow undetected into major injuries, while major injuries could become life threatening. As unpleasant as it may be, pain is an important safety mechanism designed to prevent the escalation of injury. To benefit from the messages the body sends to the brain, we must first understand them.

Traumatic physical pain may be described as an unpleasant and undesirable sensation recognized by the brain, but initiated by the irritation of pain receptor endings located throughout the body. A variety of factors at both the pain receptor level and the brain interpretation level control the manifestation of this sensation. These factors are both physical and emotional and have led to our statement that "pain, like beauty, is to some degree in the eye of the beholder."

The Significance of Injury Pain

Injury pain is a message to the brain that something is causing irritation of the nerve pain fibers. It is not always, however, an indication that serious harm is occurring. Here are some guidelines to help you differentiate harmful from non-harmful pain:

PHASES OF PAIN

BENIGN PAIN (non-harmful):
Phase 1
Stiffness or mild soreness after exercise activity. Pain is usually gone in 24 hours.

Phase 2
Stiffness or mild soreness after exercise activity which lasts beyond 48 hours. This pain is relieved by warm-up. The symptoms are not present during activity, but return after activity. This pain resolves within 72 hours without intervening exercise activity.

SEMI-BENIGN PAIN (likely non-harmful):

Phase 3

Stiffness or mild soreness before specific sport or occupational activity. Pain is partially relieved by warm-up. It is minimally present during activity and does not cause an alteration of the activity. This pain is usually controlled by precautionary activity modification and Counter-Force bracing (see Chapter IV, page 29-30). Mild anti-inflammatory medication may be indicated with Phase 3 pain. Without precautions, Phase 3 pain may progress to Phase 4.

NOTE: Exercise activity modification includes a change in sports or occupational technique, intensity, and duration, or all of these.

SEMI-HARMFUL PAIN:

Phase 4

Pain is similar to, but somewhat more intense than Phase 3 pain. Phase 4 pain causes a change in the performance of the attempted exercise activity. Mild pain may also be noticed with activities of daily living. Without precaution, Phase 4 pain could progress to Phase 5 pain. Phase 4 pain may reflect tendon damage.

HARMFUL PAIN:

Phase 5

Significant (moderate or greater) pain before, during and after exercise activity which alters activity performance, usually to the point of stopping the activity. Complete rest usually controls pain. Pain occurs with activities of daily living (ADL's), but does not cause a major change in ADL's.

Phase 5 pain usually reflects permanent tendon damage.

Phase 6

Phase 5 pain which persists even with complete rest. Phase 6 pain disrupts simple ADL's, and household chores must usually be eliminated.

Phase 7

Phase 6 pain which also causes a disruption of sleep on a consistent basis. Pain is aching in nature and intensifies with activity.

NOTE: Pain phases 5, 6 and 7 usually reflect increasing percentages of permanent tendon damage.

CAUTION: No guideline can be accurate for every individual case. If there is any question, check with your doctor. In general, however, pain Phases 1 and 2 are self-limiting with proper precaution. Phase 3 or 4 pain which persists beyond two weeks indicates the need for medical attention. Phases 5, 6 and 7 generally require medical attention.

NOTE: Although this book is primarily dedicated to the tendon problems of tennis elbow, these pain phases also have value regarding ligament and muscle injury pain.

Highlights of Chapter II

1. Pain may not always indicate harm, but should be monitored closely to differentiate harmful from non-harmful pain.

2. Pain Phases are differentiated to aid in understanding and dealing with permanent vs. non-permanent tendon damage.

Chapter III

Treatment of Injury - The Overview

The key to rehabilitation of injured tendons is restoring blood vessel supply while helping the body produce new tendon collagen protein. For return to good health, tendons must have motion, tension, blood vessel supply, oxygen and nutrition. Therefore, restoration of normal strength, endurance and flexibility are generally critical in accomplishing these healing goals. It should be appreciated that strength and endurance beyond the usual are often required if high demand sports activities are to be considered.

The basic treatment concepts of tennis elbow may be divided into six separate categories:

I. Relief of pain and chemical inflammation

II. Promotion of healing

III. Rehabilitative exercise

IV. Conditioning fitness exercise

V. Control of abusive injury producing overload activities

VI. Surgery, if conservative treatment fails

We will explore each of these areas in detail.

CAUTION: Specific treatment programs are highly individualistic. The treatment recommendations that follow are for a typical problem. It is recommended that you have the full approval, diagnosis and supervision of your doctor before implementing these treatment plans.

I. Relief of Pain and Inflammation

PRICEMM (protection, rest, ice, compression, elevation, medications, modalities)

A. Anti-inflammatory medications

Medication can be a definite aid in the treatment of tennis elbow. It is our view however that medication is not directly responsible for healing, but does aid by offering comfort. A comfortable patient is much more likely to proceed with the necessary rehabilitation procedures. Commonly used anti-inflammatory medications include aspirin, ibuprofen (brand names include Advil, Nuprin, Motrin and Rufin) and other non-steroidal anti-inflammatory medications such as Naprosyn, Ansaid, Anaprox, Dolobid, Tolectin, Clinoril, Feldene, Voltaren, Orudis, Nalfon, Indocin and others. Cortisone is also available and highly effective, but is a steroidal hormone. Our recommendation, however, is to stay on the aspirin and ibuprofen side of the medication spectrum if possible. The other mentioned medications are reserved for more special pain situations (*this includes cortisone injections*). It is recommended that all medication, including non-prescription ones, be monitored by your physician.

Cortisone injections, in our opinion, are best reserved for patients whose pain intensity is so extreme that it precludes ADL's (activities of daily living), and/or compromises the ability to proceed with the rehabilitative exercise program. Local cortisone injection can result in tissue atrophy; and therefore, no more than 3 injections are suggested if the above indications are present.

NOTE: These medicines do not promote strength, endurance, flexibility, new blood vessel supply, or new tendon protein production, they simply control the pain so that rehabilitative activities can be undertaken. They do not heal!

B. Rest

Our definition of rest is absence of abusive activity, thereby protecting the injured area from further damage; rest is *not* absence from all activity (as noted, tendons need some tension and motion to maintain their health). Total immobilization such as joint splinting or casting results in further weakness, muscle atrophy, decreased vascular demand and supply and is potentially detrimental to healing. Total rest is therefore not recommended in the usual circumstance. Rest alone does quiet pain and inflammation, but it does not necessarily encourage healing. It is critical therefore that a period of rest be followed by rehabilitative exercise to restore normal strength, endurance and flexibility (e.g., tendon health) before returning to sports or occupational participation.

NOTE: Like medication, rest does not promote strength, endurance, flexibility, new blood vessel supply, or new tendon protein production.

C. Physical Modalities
1. Ice
Ice or cold application is always advisable after injury (unless frostbite, allergic sensitivity, or poor circulation exists). Ice should be applied anytime the signs of inflammation or intense pain are present, no matter how soon or long after the injury.

Signs of inflammation:

- Swelling
- Stiffness
- Tenderness to touch
- Injured area feels feverish (warm) to touch
- Phase 3+ pain: This symptom phase suggests inflammation

Ice Can:
- Bring pain relief
- Bring spasm relief
- Reduce swelling
- Decrease inflammation

When and how to apply ice:
a. Immediately after activity or injury.
b. Place ice cubes in a plastic bag and hold to injured area with commercial Ice Strap™ or elastic wrap such as an ace bandage.
c. Use a commercial ice pack or ice cubes in a plastic bag (such as Ziplock storage bag).
   NOTE: If ice is not readily available, carry your own supply of ice cubes in a thermos jug to the activity area.
d. The duration of ice application may vary; (15-30 minutes recommended). Avoid icing for more than 30 minutes at a time as frost bite may occur. To protect skin, place a thin cloth between the ice bag and skin.
e. Ice should be used until inflammation is controlled (following a pattern of 15-30 minutes on, and 30 minutes off).

    f.   Use an ice massage.
       Ice Massage Technique: Freeze water in a dixie cup, tear paper until ice is
       exposed, massage over inflamed area for 5 minutes. May repeat every 20-
       30 minutes if pain returns.

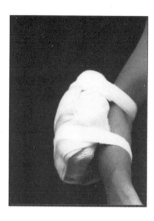

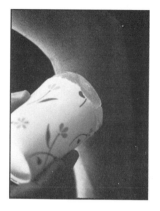

Ice Strap™

Ice Massage

NOTE: It often takes days, and sometimes weeks, before full inflammation control is achieved and ice may be indicated on an intermittent basis for this entire time.

CAUTION: If excessive skin redness from ice applications occurs, check with your doctor. Do not use ice if frostbite, hardening of the arteries, poor circulation, or sensitivity to cold is present or has occurred in the past.

   2. Heat
      Heat application also relieves pain and spasm, but has the potential to increase
      swelling and inflammation. Thus, heat is indicated in the early stages of injury
      only under the following conditions:

      a. if used as a warm-up before exercise
      b. if followed by ice application
      c. if signs of inflammation have been eliminated

      NOTE: Heat can be applied in many forms including hot showers, electric
      pad and moist heat. Moist heat by hydrocollator, whirlpool or
      thermophore pad are generally the most effective.

Recipe for Microwave hot packs
Method:
1. Place a towel under warm tap water, then wring it out.
2. Fold towel in half 3 times.
3. Place towel in open Ziplock bag.
4. Place bag in microwave oven set on high setting for 2 minutes.
5. Remove hot pack from oven; wrap it with dry toweling.
6. Cover body part with amount of toweling needed to avoid burning, while keeping the area as warm as possible.

Materials:
One 10 9/16" x 11" Ziplock storage bag
One 18" x 34" white bath towel
Adapted from: CLINICAL MANAGEMENT, VOL. 6, NO. 3
Peter Degere, PT, Mercy Hospital, 1000 N. Village Ave., RVC, New York 11570.

The duration of heat application varies, dependent upon the intensity and type of heat application. Low intensity heat such as a heat lamp or pad on low may be well tolerated and comforting for an hour or more. Exposure to high intensity heat such as a hot hydrocollator is best restricted to 20 minutes or less.

Caution: Application of hot packs can result in burning. Check skin carefully during treatment.

3. Ultrasound
   Ultrasound is a deep-heat modality, in which heat is generated by sound waves as they are absorbed by deep tissue. It is generally not effective in treating tennis elbow in our experience. If used at the elbow, water inter-face is preferable to gel.

4. High Voltage Electrical Stimulation
   This modality is effective in reducing pain and stiffness, enhancing blood flow and controlling inflammation. We have found this to be the most effective physical therapy modality in treating tennis elbow.

   NOTE: High voltage stimulation should not be confused with transcutaneous nerve stimulation (TNS) which is a superficial skin nerve stimulator.

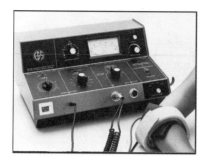

High Voltage Electrical Stimulator

5. Other Physical Therapy Modalities

   Other techniques available for physical therapy treatment include phonophoresis (ultrasound with cortisone cream), and iontophoresis (electrical stimulation with corticosteroid/anesthetic lotion). The addition of cortisone cream, in our experience,offers no additional benefit over the standard properly applied high voltage electrical stimulation and may have the same potential harmful side effects of other cortisone treatments.

6. Compression Techniques

   For arm swelling (which is often noted after competitive baseball pitching), the use of a graduated air compression sleeve unit, which mechanically squeezes the extra fluid out of the extremity, has been helpful.

7. Deep friction massage

   Some physical therapists have reported occasional success with the use of a deep massaging technique or manipulation of the sensitive areas. Our experience at Virginia Sportsmedicine Institute has not supported these techniques as offering any advantage in the usual case of tennis elbow. In addition, these techniques tend to be painful, making compliance with the exercise programs difficult.

8. Changing technology

   Medical technology is changing rapidly and we look forward to further advances and successes in using the modalities of physical therapy.

9. Unorthodox Methods

   Acupuncture and DSMO application are occasionally cited by patients as helpful. We have prescribed neither, but have treated many patients who have admitted to receiving or have self-applied such treatments. In our discussion with these patients neither treatment has demonstrated any benefits other than occasional short term pain relief (a few weeks at most), possibly by placebo effect. There has been no observed evidence of increased strength or elimination of the pathological damage in tendon or muscle tissue by use of these methods.

NOTE: If the treatment had been curative, the patients would not have been in need of further care!

II. Promotion of Healing

The promotion of healing is separate and distinct from pain relief. The enhancement of healing requires new blood vessel supply, organization and strengthening of healing body protein (collagen), plus the promotion of strength, endurance and flexibility in the injured and adjacent tissue.

When pain is reduced so that ADL's are comfortable and no local heat is noted at the injured area, the limbering exercises and follow-up treatments below may be started. **NOTE:** The pain relief offered from a cortisone injection may confuse this determination.

A. Active motion exercises to the injured areas (e.g. motion done by you the patient).
   NOTE: Passive stretching may cause further tissue injury and is not usually recommended (e.g., stretching done by another person or machine).

These exercises are best done after warming the elbow and wrist in warm water or with a heating pad, or after general body warm-up exercises. General active warm-up to the point of sweating is best. Jumpings jacks, arm circles, or arm cycling are excellent techniques for active warm-up (see Chapter V, pg. 36).

Active elbow and forearm flexibility exercises:
   1. Actively bend and stretch the elbow fully,
   2. With the elbow bent at the side, turn the palm up, then down,
   3. With the elbow bent at the side, palm down and hand gently closed, bend wrist back, then down,
   4. Open all fingers widely and close with elbow bent at the side
   Repeat each exercise 5 - 10 times, up to 5 times a day.

B. Continue use of high voltage electrical stimulation on a selective basis to control pain and inflammation and enhance new blood vessel supply.

C. Ice for 15 - 30 minutes after exercise. Once full active motion becomes comfortable and there is no pain with these exercises or ADL's, rehabilitative resistance exercises can begin.

III. General Concepts of Rehabilitative Exercises to Promote Healing, Strength and Endurance

Rehabilitative resistance exercises are specifically designed to stimulate healing of the injured tissue. As such, the exercise programs are quite precise and specific. These exercises are usually best done under the supervision of a medical professional (e.g., your physician or licensed physical therapist). Ideally, you should undergo baseline strength tests of the injured and non-injured arms to quantify strength deficits and establish exercise end points.

A. Baseline strength test
To understand the magnitude of strength deficits and assess the effectiveness of the exercise program, it is essential to have some form of strength test and a measurement of atrophy. Isokinetic dynamometer (such as Cybex testing machines) offers a highly sophisticated strength test, and is the ideal. A practical, less detailed clinical form of measurement is the grip strength dynamometer.

NOTE: Weakness is often present throughout the entire arm including shoulder and upper back, as well as, the painful areas around the elbow.

B. Circumferential Measurement
A quick and effective test to determine atrophy and compare the injured to the uninjured arm is to measure the circumference of the forearm at the point just below the elbow. The normal dominant forearm usually measures 1/4 inch greater in males and 1/8 inch greater in females. In highly competitive racquet and throwing sport athletes this differential is usually greater (up to 1 1/4 inches in world class athletes).

Goals of Rehabilitation

The overall purpose of the rehabilitative exercise program for the injured elbow tendons is to restore new blood vessel supply in association with restoration of strength, endurance and flexibility to a normal or above normal level The muscle-tendon units involved in tennis elbow originate just above the elbow joint. They act to turn the palm up and down, to bend the wrist up and down, and to open and close the fingers.

If the stated goals can be accomplished, permanent pain relief almost always follows.

Protections During Resistance Exercise

To guard against exercise overload and provide comfort during resistance exercises we recommend:

1. Supervision of the program by a physician or licensed physical therapist.

2. Count'R-Force® Bracing
    Lateral or Medial elbow bracing (depending on the type of tennis elbow) is recommended during the first 3-4 weeks of the rehabilitative program while doing the exercises and during the entire time of treatment when the arm is used repetitively or aggressively during the ADL's. Examples of such activities include typing, writing, carpentry (e.g., hammering or use of screw driver), carrying packages, cleaning, cooking and the like.

3. Controlling inflammation
    If your doctor approves, take two buffered aspirin or one ibuprofen 15 to 30 minutes before rehabilitative exercise. This helps to relieve stiffness and control the potential for inflammation which can occur with rehabilitative exercise. In special circumstances, your doctor may elect to use a stronger prescription anti-inflammatory medication.

4. Warmers
    If additional warmth is comforting, especially during cold weather, an elbow warmer can easily be constructed by cutting the toe out of an old wool sock and pulling it over the Count'R-Force® brace at the elbow. Commercial warmers of wool or orlon (easily obtained at retail dance or exercise shops) are quite inexpensive, comfortable and effective.

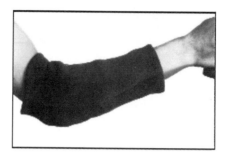

Use of a warmer in cool
environments aids in the comfort and
implementation of the exercises.

IV. Conditioning Fitness Exercise

It is important to note that lack of normal activities has a detrimental physical and mental effect. A tunnel vision approach of only concentrating on the injured area is, in our view, a poor one. Overall a "domino effect" leading to weakness of adjacent uninjured areas occurs quickly (e.g., the entire arm, shoulder, neck, and upper back often weaken) in association with tennis elbow. This weakness must be prevented or eliminated because secondary injury to these other tissues can occur (such as shoulder tendinitis). In addition, full body aerobic and muscle conditioning is easily lost and fat weight gain may occur. For these reasons, we recommend that an aggressive, overall conditioning program be started as early as possible.

It should be noted that conditioning exercise is quite different from rehabilitative exercise, although each may enhance the effectiveness of the other. The higher intensity of the conditioning programs is designed for essentially normal or uninjured tissue. Care should be taken to ensure, therefore, that these body parts called into play during these exercises are not weak or injured. Examination by your doctor may be needed to determine this. If injured tissue is subjected to conditioning exercise without first being rehabilitated, further damage may occur.

Exercise to *uninjured areas* can be instituted at any time after elbow injury occurs (the sooner, the better) so long as the *injured areas* are not subject to excessive force during the conditioning exercise program. In upper extremity injury, maintenance of aerobic conditioning, leg and back strength and flexibility can often be attained by running, biking, using strength machines, etc. Body parts adjacent to the injured area should also be exercised early (such as neck and shoulder). In fact, exercise to these adjacent areas may well stimulate the healing process in the injured elbow tissue by nutritional and oxygenation enhancement to the entire extremity. In addition, fitness exercise is a wonderful way to counteract the detrimental emotional effects often associated with injury.

V. Control of Abusive Injury Producing Overload Activities

The principles of overload control are covered in Chapter IV. The outline of these principles include:

A. Count'R-Force® bracing
B. Control of intensity and duration of activities
C. Technique modification
D. Protective equipment
E. Size and type of sport or occupational equipment for performance and good health
F. Appropriate grip size for implement activities (e.g. tennis racquet handle, etc.)

VI. Surgery

The concepts of surgery are covered in Chapter VII. In general, surgery is considered only if a quality rehabilitative effort fails. We must emphasize, however, that the program of rehabilitation must be a quality program which focuses on active resistance exercise which is methodically progressed. Each patient's program must be carefully individualized to meet his or her specific needs, goals, and rehabilitation potential. It has been our observation that many sessions of physical therapy which emphasize comfort are inadequate to accomplish the necessary goals of rehabilitation. Thus weeks or months of "comfort" physical therapy, or passive physical therapy (e.g., rest, modalities, stretching, and massage) without true rehabilitative exercise are usually ineffective. Prior to considering surgery, therefore, we often find it appropriate to reinstitute a meaningful physical therapy rehabilitation program. It is, of course, best if an appropriate program is instituted from the start.

Highlights of Chapter III

1. The concepts of treatment include:
   a. Relief of pain
   b. Promotion of healing
   c. Rehabilitative resistance exercise
   d. Fitness exercise
   e. Control of abusive activities
   f. Surgery

2. The goals of treatment are to heal injured tendon tissue by encouraging new blood vessel and collagen protein formation, as well as, restoring strength, endurance and flexibility to normal levels. This is best accomplished by rehabilitative resistance exercises with the aid of measures which provide comfort.

3. Isolated use of rest and anti-inflammatory medications may comfort, but they do not directly heal or strengthen injured tissue.

Chapter IV

Control of Injury Producing Overuse

Tendon injury may be caused by a single stress event or the build up of many smaller stress events which eventually cause a tendon to give out. The build up of these stress events is known as injury producing overuse or abusive overload. Control of this overload is vital to maintain healthy activity levels.

The principles of controlling abusive overload include:
A. Counter-Force bracing
B. Modification of intensity, duration and technique of forearm activity
C. Use of the proper size and type of equipment for both performance and protection. These principles and concepts are equally appropriate for the prevention of injury and for injury rehabilitation.

We have found the principles for the control of abuse extremely beneficial during these phases of rehabilitation:

1. Rest phase
2. Early phases of rehabilitative resistance exercise
3. Fitness exercise
4. ADL's requiring aggressive forearm use
5. Return to sports or occupational activities

In general, the principles of abusive overuse control are used in a mix that is dependent upon the variables of the magnitude of injury, fitness level, strength deficits, and the nature of occupational or sports activities.

A. Counter-Force bracing
   The term counter-force as applied to bracing was introduced by the senior author (R.P.N.) in 1972. Its principle is to give firm, but pliable anatomical support and protection for an expanding muscle or moving tendon, while at the same time allowing freedom of joint movement. In our observations, braces which block joint motion or apply pressure to small areas are less effective and possibly troublesome. The blocking of joint motion invites atrophy and muscle weakness while small area compression invites muscle imbalance and the potential of excess focal compression.

The pulling or expanding of a contracting muscle-tendon unit is theorized to gently push off the counter-force brace, thereby decreasing internal muscle tension and lending needed support to injured tendons without pinching blood vessels or nerves. The Count'R-Force® braces utilized at Virginia Sportsmedicine Institute were designed by the senior author (R.P.N.), two tension straps for the lateral and three for the medial tennis elbow brace have proven best. The most effective clinical design, in our observations, include the following characteristics: 2 3/4" wide; curved to fit the conical shape of the forearm, and multiple tension straps for complete brace control. We have noted that evenly balanced circumferential compression maintains the comfortable muscle balance so important to the rehabilitation process. Count'R-Force® braces (lateral elbow, medial elbow and wrist) have proven highly successful in pain relief. Biomechanical and nerve conduction studies have demonstrated the beneficial actions of the Count'R-Force® braces (e.g., decreased angular acceleration at the elbow and decreased muscle activity). Counter-force braces should be utilized only during the time of potentially injurious activity or at the start of rehabilitative exercise.

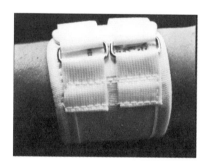 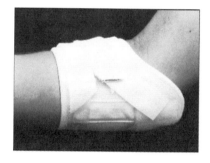

Lateral Count'R-Force®
Tennis Elbow Brace

Medial Count'R-Force®
Tennis Elbow Brace

Photos courtesy Medical Sports, Inc. Arlington, Virginia

Wide, anatomically designed, non-elastic braces, with multiple tension straps for balanced muscle support and full patient control, offer ideal counter-force control.

NOTE: The desirable duration of counter-force use during rehabilitation exercise is highly individualistic. Usual durations are four to six weeks after the start of rehabilitation exercise. For sports activity, Counter-force braces should be used as a protective precaution.

B. Control of intensity and duration of forearm use:
In this category, pain is a very helpful guide. It is our recommendation that the pain phases as noted in Chapter II be adhered to as a reasonable approach to monitoring the potential for activity overload. If pain phase IV is reached, modification of sports, occupation, fitness, or rehabilitative exercise is critical.

C. Forearm Technique Modification (sports or occupation):
In Chapter I several illustrations concerning sport technique were offered. It is clear that the techniques of many activities (occupational, sports and ADL's) can cause injurious overload. It has been our experience that many techniques can be altered or modified to protect the arm and still be highly effective for sport or occupational performance. We strongly recommend, therefore, that an analysis of sport or occupation technique by knowledgeable medical specialists, coaches, biomechanists or occupational supervisors be undertaken and that changes to eliminate potentially injurious techniques be made where necessary.

D. Protective Equipment or Occupational Environment:

   1. Overview
   It is quite clear that equipment size, design and material can and do affect injury potential by either increasing or decreasing abusive forces. It is important to analyze the equipment used and the ergonomics of the work place, sport, or performing arts environment.

   2. Examples of Equipment Choices
   In tennis, the present clinical experience at the Nirschl Orthopedic/ Sportsmedicine Clinic and Virginia Sportsmedicine Institute in regard to tennis racquets suggest the following guidelines for best protection against injury. It should be noted that torsion control, not vibration control, appears to be a more important factor in controlling abusive forces.

      a. Racquet Size
      Mid-sized (90 -110 square inch hitting zone)

      b. Frame Materials
      Graphite should be the major component. No identifiable clinical differences have been noted concerning additional percentages of other materials (e.g., Boron, Kevlar, Ceramic, etc.)

c. Frame Contour
No identifiable advantages or disadvantages have been noted (e.g., flat ends, oval shape, etc.)

d. Frame Flexibility (wide and standard bodies)
Medium flex racquets appear the most benevolent. In this context, wide body designs are generally stiffer and may, in theory, be *more* troublesome. Non-scientific clinical observation seems to confirm the potential for greater overuse symptoms with wide body racquets.

e. String Tension
We recommend stringing the racquet at the lowest tension range recommended by the manufacturer of the racquet chosen. Lower string tensions have been noted to be more comfortable.

f. String Type
Quality mono-filament nylon is durable and consistent and seems best overall. Gut strings may be more forgiving when new, but deteriorate rapidly and would require frequent expensive restringing to maintain any advantage.

g. Anti-Vibration Devices
Some symptomatic patients report pain control with devices attached to the strings, but the evidence for major benefit is not compelling. As noted above, torsion control rather than vibration control appears to be the key factor in tennis elbow prevention and treatment concerning tennis racquets.

3. Grip size for hand held implements subject to twisting motions.
A small grip creates a torsion leverage disadvantage inviting a high probability of forearm muscle-tendon overload (e.g., symptomatic tennis elbow).

Look at the palm of the hand. Notice the palmar creases. Using a ruler, (see illustration p. 33) measure from the bottom crease (running along the middle portion of your hand between the long and ring finger), to the tip of your ring finger. This determines the grip you need. For example if the measurement is 4 1/2 inches, that is the best grip size for you.

4. Example of work place environment
In the computer office setting the design of the computer key board, the monitor height and height of computer desk often result in forearm overload and tennis elbow (see illustration p. 33).

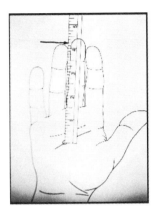

Hand size measurement. Nirschl Technique.
For tennis racquets and other hand held implements.

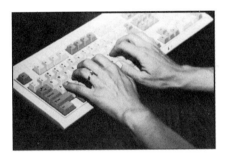

Height of computer key board affects wrist position and potential for forearm
muscle-tendon overload. A flat keyboard which decreases the backward angle
of the wrist (eg. less dorsi-flexion) is best.

Highlights of Chapter IV

1. Abusive overload activities cause injury (e.g., overuse).
2. Control of abusive overload includes:
   a. Monitoring intensity and duration of activities
   b. Changing poor activity techniques
   c. Count'R-Force® bracing
   d. Using proper equipment including proper grip size

Chapter V

Warm-Up

Exercise warm-up is an important part of any work-out routine. The warm-up prepares the muscles and connective tissue for the more rigorous demands of the work-out. When injured tissue is involved, the warm-up takes on an added importance.

Muscles and tendons are intertwined with lard-like substances called extra-cellular ground substance. When this substance gels, its consistency becomes like that of lard in a refrigerator, resulting in stiffness and extra tissue friction during motion. A gentle pre-activity or pre-exercise period of warm-up (until a light sweat occurs) will prepare your muscles, tendons, ligaments and joints for a relaxed, comfortable exercise program. This internal warm-up heats the gelled substance reducing stiffness and friction and preparing the body for the rigors of the work-out. If a specific body part is stiff, you may begin your warm-up with passive external warming (e.g. such as that provided by a heating pad, or warm water immersion such as whirlpool, sauna, or hot shower). Following this technique, massage the stiff or sore area with a methyl salicylate product such as Craemergesic or Ben-Gay. Next, apply the appropriate Count'R-Force® elbow brace, and in cold environments, an overlaying joint warmer. Finally, proceed with an active internal warm-up. This active exercise warm-up is preferable to a passive external warm-up because the big muscles of the body generate heat which is deep and long lasting. If time is a problem, passive heating (external warm-up) may be eliminated from the warm-up routine, but do not eliminate the active warm-up exercises.

Proper internal warm-up also prepares your heart for more aggressive activity. Without gradual warm-up, sudden intense exercise often results in missed heart beats which could be dangerous. *CAUTION: STRETCHING OR FLEXIBILITY EXER-CISE DOES NOT CONSTITUTE A WARM-UP.* In fact, stretching before warm-up exercise invites injury because the cooled ground substances are less pliable and a friction effect is created for gliding muscles and tendons. Warm-up before stretching allows a smooth, lubricated gliding effect which results in more pliable tissues.

Warm-up check list:
1. Take two buffered aspirin or ibuprofen, with doctor's approval, thirty minutes before activity if needed to aid in controlling stiffness.
2. At your discretion, apply passive external warming to stiff areas.
3. Massage sore or stiff areas.
4. Apply the appropriate Count'R-Force* elbow brace to protect injured tendons.
5. Apply joint warmer in a cool environment.
6. Do warm-up exercises until a light sweat occurs.
7. Follow warm-up with flexibility exercise as appropriate (check with a medical professional).
8. Follow with rehabilitative, fitness, or sports exercise as indicated.

Active Internal Warm-up Exercises

Any gradual activity which uses the large central body muscles is a proper warm-up technique. Passive external warming may be helpful; but, active exercise is best since the warming is deeper, more extensive, and gets the muscles and heart involved. Good techniques include running in place, performing jumping jacks, briskly walking, jogging, bicycling (stationary or road bicycling) and light calisthenics until a light sweat occurs. Usually 3-5 minutes are needed for warm-up. Warm-ups for the arms include shoulder shrugs, arm swings or arm cycling.

Warm-up Techniques

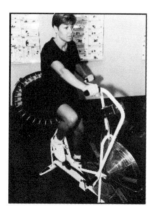

Schwinn Airdyne

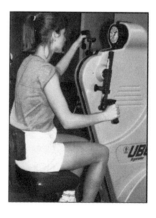

Cybex Arm Cycle (U.B.E.)

Flexibility Exercise

As noted, flexibility or stretching exercises do not replace a warm-up. Stretching cold and stiff tissues subject tendons, muscles, and joints to high friction forces and invites injury. Flexibility exercise should be done only after a proper warm-up.

In addition, it has been our experience that the majority of exercise enthusiasts do not have accurate goals or proper reasons for stretching. The reasons for flexibility programs are highly individualistic and the techniques are precise. We recommend that you check with your doctor or physical therapist for specific recommendations.

Rehabilitative Strength Exercises

Following proper warm-up, appropriate strengthening exercises can be under-taken. In the early phases of healing, these exercises involve minimal resistance and high repetition to stimulate the early healing process without risking further tissue damage. As healing progresses, the program gradually shifts to higher resistances (weights, etc.) and fewer repetitions.

Highlights of Chapter V

1. Warm-up and flexibility exercise are separate and distinct. Stretching should not be done without proper warm-up (e.g. while the body is still cold).

2. Warm-up can be either external passive or internal active. Internal active warm-up is best.

3. Warm-up should always be done prior to flexibility, rehabilitative, fitness or sports exercise.

Chapter VI

Rehabilitative Exercise Program

The rehabilitative exercise program is the key component in healing the chronic damage of tendinitis/tendinosis (medical term is angio-fibroblastic tendinosis). The goal of the program is to promote healing by:

1. Encouraging new blood vessel supply (collateral circulation) thereby enhancing nutrition and oxygenation to the damaged tissue. One might describe this as "aerobic exercise for tendons."
2. Encouraging the formation of healing tissue cells (fibroblasts) and healing materials such as the protein collagen and extra-cellular ground substances.
3. Organizing the biological alignment of the healing tissue fibers for proper strength and function.
4. Strengthening and maturing the newly formed tissue to accept the high stresses of sports or occupational activities.

Accomplishing the goals of biological healing requires precision and perseverance. Medical supervision by your physician or physical therapist ensures the best result.

General Exercise Principles

1. These exercises can be useful not only for rehabilitation, but also as a forearm conditioning program to prevent injury and enhance the performance of such upper extremity activities as tennis, baseball, squash, racquetball, golf, performing arts (piano, percussion and string instruments), and many occupational activities.

2. If you have a known problem with the elbow or wrist, this program is to be undertaken only with your physician's approval.
    a. Do not start the exercise program until normal pain-free motion of the elbow and wrist have been achieved.
    b. Do not start this exercise program until pain relief has been achieved when doing ADL's.

3. Maintain your overall fitness level. When you are recovering from any injury, it is essential for you to:

   a. Maintain your cardiovascular (heart/lung) fitness level through aerobic exercise. The key ingredient of any aerobic exercise program is sustained effort. It is generally agreed by physicians versed in sports medicine that a convenient and accurate assessment of heart/lung work can be obtained by measuring the pulse rate. It is further agreed that twenty minutes of sustained effort three times per week, at an intensity of seventy percent of maximum pulse rate, is the "minimum effort" required for a reasonable state of heart/lung fitness. Increased effort over the minimum increases the fitness level.

Target (exercise) heart rate (THR) determination

220 - age = maximum heart rate (MHR)

THR = 80% of MHR.

Example of 40-year-old:

220 - 40 = 180 MHR

180 x 80% = 144 THR

   b. Maintain and/or improve strength, flexibility and endurance of the other body areas. Tennis elbow is often directly attributable to deficits in the shoulder, trunk and legs (for example, poor tennis technique results if you get to the ball late because of leg deficiencies). These deficiencies may be present from old injuries that never fully rehabilitated or from subtle, undetected hereditary deficiencies. This is an excellent time to correct these deficits.

   c. Maintain your agility level by use of agility drills such as the hexagon or Carioca side movement drills.

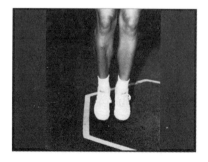 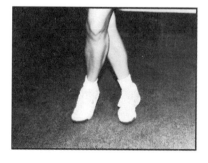

Hexagon Agility Drill   Carioca Movement Agility Drill

Overview of Rehabilitative Strength Program

The rehabilitative strength program is vital to full recovery. The program consists of a precise progression through multiple resistance systems including Isotonic (weight), Isoflex (tension cord), Isometric (internal muscle tension) and the Isokinetic (hydraulic fixed speed). This progression has been developed by our clinical observations of thousands of patients and has proven the best over many observed sequences. Prior to starting the exercise program, we recommend you keep the following points in mind.

1. Before beginning strengthening exercise, warm-up the body to a light sweat (3-5 minutes of brisk walking, cycling, jogging, etc.). In addition, warm the injured area with passive external heat (heat pad, hotwater bottle, etc.).
2. A gradual progression is extremely important to prevent re-aggravation of symptoms and inflammation.
3. Wear the appropriate Count'R-Force® brace (check with your physician or therapist regarding duration).
4. Ice the elbow for 20-30 minutes after exercise if any swelling, stiffness, soreness or pain is present.

Isotonic exercises (to 3 pounds)

The isotonic exercises (wrist flexion, wrist extension, forearm rotations) are described on the following pages. For all three exercises, follow these guidelines for progression. Keep elbow *bent* 90° with the forearm well supported on your thigh or a table. Begin with no weight and perform 15-20 repetitions daily. Once you can comfortably do 20 repetitions for 2 consecutive sessions, add 1 pound and go back to 15 repetitions. Work up to 20 repetitions. Once you can comfortably do the 20 repetitions with 1 pound for 2 consecutive sessions, increase the weight to 2 pounds, cut back to 15 repetitions and again progress to 20 repetitions. Once you are comfortably performing 20 repetitions with 2 pounds for 2 consecutive sessions, increase weight to 3 pounds, do 12 repetitions and work up to 15 repetitions with the 3 pounds.

Do each exercise at its own rate. You will achieve higher weights on some exercises than on others.

Do each exercise with proper form: 2 seconds to raise, 2 seconds hold, 2 seconds to lower.

Isometric exercises (tennis ball squeeze & rubber band exercises):

Begin isometric exercises at the same time as the start of the isotonic program. Begin with elbow bent at side; over time progress to doing exercises with elbow straightened . The isometric program with elbow straight usually begins at the time of elbow straightening with the isotonic program (see next section, Isotonic Progression). Do these exercises frequently throughout the day every day. It's a good idea to have a tennis ball and rubber band in convenient places (such as in your car, at your desk, or by the telephone).

DO NOT CAUSE PAIN !!!
If an exercise causes Phase 4 pain, or more, modify by:
a. Decreasing weight and/or
b. Decreasing repetitions and/or
c. Going through a lesser range of motion. If it is still painful, check with your physical therapist.

Isotonic Functional Progression

Once comfortably doing 15 repetitions for 2 consecutive sessions with 3 pounds, gradually work toward straightening elbow, arm unsupported (elbow straight but not locked). When comfortable with 3 pounds doing 15 repetitions with the elbow straight, begin *alternate days* with Iso'-Flex® exercise resistance.* On the days when exercising with weights, progress to weight end point (see table) by increasing the weight by 1 pound starting at 12 repetitions. Each time you are comfortably doing 2 consecutive sessions of 15 repetitions continue progression.

Average Maximum End Points (male & female)

Exercise	M	F
wrist flexor curls	9 lbs.	6 lbs.
wrist extensor curls	7 lbs.	5 lbs.
forearm rotations	10 lbs.	8 lbs.

Continue to do the Isometric Program (eg. tennis ball and rubber band exercises) every day, throughout the day.

*Iso'-Flex® Program

Once able to do 3 pounds, 15 repetitions comfortably on a daily basis with the isotonic (weight) exercises with elbow straight, repeat weight exercises every other day as described above, alternating with the Iso'-Flex® program (e.g., 3 days of isotonic exercise and 3 days of Iso'-Flex® exercise, and 1 day of rest per week). Begin with 5 repetitions on each Iso'-Flex® exercise, and progress as indicated. See section on Iso'-Flex® Program Specifics.

The reason to utilize multiple resistance systems is that it enhances the results of treatment. Each resistance system actually exercises the muscle-tendon unit in a different manner which stimulates the healing of these tissues.

I. Isotonic Exercises (Technique Specifics)

1. Flexor Wrist Curls: (Flexors - Medial Elbow)
    A. Exercise Benefit: Forearm Flexors
    B. Starting Position: Sit in chair, elbow bent to 90° with forearm resting on table or thigh, wrist and hand extending past edge of table or thigh. Hold weight with palm up and wrist stretched down.
    C. Starting Weight: 0 pounds, progress as indicated. End point usually 6 pounds for females, 9 pounds for males.

Isotonic Flexor Wrist Curls

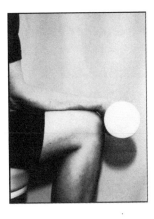 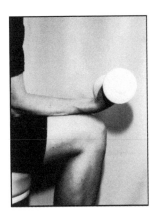

Starting Position   Exercise Action

D. Exercise Action:
   Phase 1- Slowly lift hand (flex wrist) as high as possible and hold for 2 seconds. *Keep forearm on table or thigh.*
   Phase 2- Slowly return to starting position. Repeat action and exercise progression (noted in instructions section Isotonic Exercises).
   Phase 3- (Optional) Repeat phases one and two with opposite arm.
E. Proceed to Isotonic Functional Progression (see page 42).

2. Extensor Wrist Curl: (Extensors - Lateral Elbow)
   A. Exercise Benefit: Forearm extensors
   B. Starting Position: Sit in chair, elbow bent to 90° forearm resting on table or thigh, wrist and hand extending past edge of table or thigh. Hold weight with palm down and wrist stretched down.
   C. Starting Weight: 0 pounds, progress as indicated. End points are usually 5 pounds for females and 7 pounds for males.

Isotonic Extensor Wrist Curls

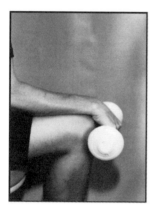 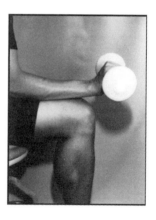

Starting Position   Exercise Action

D. Exercise Action:
   Phase 1- Slowly lift hand as high as possible and hold for 2 seconds. Maintain forearm on the thigh or table.
   Phase 2- Slowly return to starting position. Repeat action and exercise progression as noted in instruction section Isotonics exercises (to 3 pounds) (see page 41)
   Phase 3- (Optional) Repeat phases one and two with opposite arm.

E.   Proceed to Isotonic Functional Progression (see instructions on page 42).

3.   Forearm Rotations:
     A.   Exercise Benefit: Forearm pronators and supinators.
     B.   Starting Position: Sit in chair or stand with feet comfortably apart. Hold dumbbell in front of body with elbow bent to 90°. Forearm supinated (palm up).
     C.   Starting Weight: 0 pounds, progress as indicated. End points usually 8 pounds for females and 10 pounds for males.

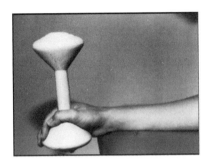

Isotonic Forearm Rotation

     D.   ExerciseAction:
          Phase 1- Slowly roll forearm to full pronated (palm down) position, then return to starting position.
          Phase 2- Repeat action and exercise progression as noted in Instructions Section (Isotonics to 3 pounds).
          Phase 3- (Optional) Repeat phase one and two with opposite arm.
     E.   Proceed to Isotonic Functional Progression (see instructions on page 42).
     F.   **NOTE:** A dumbbell with weight on one end is more effective for rotational exercise. End point of exercise weight may need to be decreased when uni-weighted dumbell is utilized.

Uni-weight:

Uni-weight is essentially a dumbbell on only one end. A twelve inch handle allows increasing leverage as the uni-weight is held further from the weighted end. This system increases the efficiency of rotational exercise. By using the leverage principle, a smaller selection of weights are needed (usually a 1, 2, 3 and 4 pound uni-weight are all that are needed for the average recreational athlete). Substitutes could include common household items such as a hammer. The length of the lever (distance from weight to the end of the handle) varies from 1 to 8 inches. The longer the lever the more difficult the exercise.

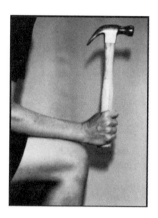

Uni-weight Substitute:
common household hammer

II. Iso'-Flex® Exercises - Overview

The exercises described are for injury rehabilitation, but Iso'-Flex® exercises can also be used as a fitness tool.* Physical therapists can improvise with other rubber band or surgical tubing materials, but a resistance system with a comfortable handle encourages good exercise compliance.

Iso'-Flex® exercise is started when each exercise of the isotonic weight program has progressed comfortably to 15 repetitions of 3 pounds with the elbow straight. The Iso'-Flex® (variable speed, variable resistance) is an evenly controlled resistance by a flexible

---

* Nirschl, R.P.: Iso'-Flex® Exercise System. Arlington, Virginia, Medical Sports, Inc. Publishing, 1982.

exercise tension cord. The exercise intensity is totally controlled by the exerciser but the resistance can be quite demanding.

Although the motions of some of the Iso'-Flex® exercises in this program are similar to the isotonic program, the resistance delivered is quite different. For example, the resistance of the Iso'-Flex® is greatest in the hold positions of the exercise; whereas, the resistance is the least with isotonic weights. The Iso'-Flex® program also adds other exercises (such as radial and ulnar deviation).

Alternate Iso'-Flex® and isotonic exercises on an every other day schedule (example: Iso'-Flex® on Mon., Wed., Fri., Isotonics on Tues., Thurs., Sat.).

Isoflex Techniques

1. Begin with 5 repetitions through the full motion described. Increase by one to two repetitions, plateau at that number of repetitions for 2-3 exercise sessions then proceed on a gradual basis until 25 repetitions are reached..
2. Do each exercise slowly and to proper form: raise 2 seconds, hold 2 seconds, lower 2 seconds.
3. Record your progress on the enclosed record.
4. Breathe normally.
5. If Phase 4 pain occurs, you are progressing at too fast a pace. Proceed with exercise modifications.**

   **Exercise Modifications:*

   The Iso'-Flex® exercise intensity can be decreased by:
   a. Doing less repetitions.
   b. Going through a partial range of motion only (e.g., non-painful range), or using the uninvolved hand to assist through the painful range.
   c. Doing "negatives" or eccentric exercise: use the opposite uninvolved hand to help raise the wrist, then lower with only the involved hand working.
6. Once you can comfortably do 25 repetitions of an Iso'-Flex® exercise, replace the slow repetitions with anaerobic sprints. (See Anaerobic Sprints, next section).

Iso'-Flex® Technique - Caution:

CAUTION: The Iso'-Flex® must be secure to prevent elastic recoil which could strike your body. Keep Iso'-Flex® firmly attached or stabilized under your foot at all times and do not pull toward your face or eyes.

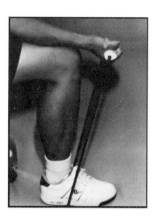

Keep Iso'-Flex® firmly attached or stabilized under your foot at all times.

Iso'-Flex® Exercise - Technique Specifics

1. Flexor Wrist Curls:
   A. Exercise Benefit: Forearm flexors
   B. Starting Position: Sit in chair and place Iso'-Flex® *firmly* under your right foot. Hold handle in your right hand, palm up. With elbow bent at 90°, support forearm on thigh with wrist and hand extended just beyond right knee.

Iso'-Flex® Flexor Wrist Curls

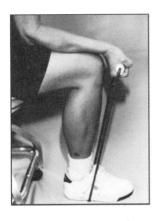

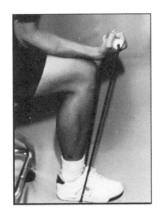

Starting Position   Exercise Action

C. Exercise Action:
   Phase 1- From wrist-back (extended position), slowly curl
   wrist up. Hold firmly for 2-3 seconds.
   Phase 2- Slowly return to starting position. Repeat 5 times. Progress
   slowly to 25 repetitions.
   Phase 3- Repeat phases one and two with left arm if indicated,
   Iso'-Flex® *firmly* under left foot.
   Phase 4- Anaerobic sprints - Progress to anaerobic sprints
   after 25 at normal speed repetitions can be performed with comfort (see
   pages 56-57).

2. Radial Wrist Curls:
   A. Exercise Benefit: Radial wrist extensors, wrist adductors
   B. Starting Position: Sit in chair and place Iso'-Flex® *firmly* under your
      right foot. Hold handle in your right hand with thumb knuckle and Iso'-
      Flex® handle end pointing up. With elbow bent, support forearm on
      thigh with wrist and hand extended just beyond right knee.

Iso'-Flex® Radial Wrist Curls

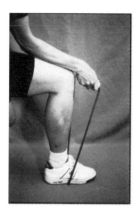

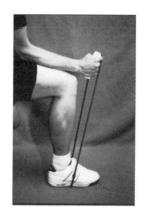

Starting Position   Exercise Action

C. Exercise Action:

Phase 1- Lift hand up toward forearm as high as possible. Hold *firmly* for 2 seconds.

Phase 2- Return slowly to starting position. Repeat 5 times. Progress slowly to 25 repetitions.

Phase 3- Repeat phases one and two with left arm if indicated, Iso'-Flex® firmly under left foot.

Phase 4- Anaerobic sprints - Progress to anaerobic sprints after 25 repetitions at normal speed can be completed comfortably (see pages 56-57).

3. Forearm Pronation:
   A. Exercise Benefit: Forearm pronators
   B. Starting Position: Sit in chair and place Iso'-Flex® firmly under your left foot. Left foot should be positioned ten inches outside center of body. Hold handle in you right hand with palm up. With elbow bent, support forearm on thigh with wrist and hand extended just beyond right knee.

Iso'-Flex® Forearm Pronation

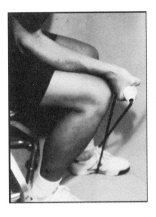

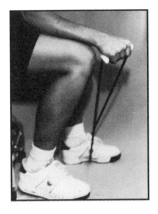

Starting Position

Exercise Action

C. Exercise Action:

Phase 1- Slowly rotate forearm to palm down position, right hand index finger knuckle pointing to inside of left knee. Hold firmly for 2 seconds.

Phase 2- Slowly return to starting position. Repeat 5 times. Progress slowly to 25 repetitions.

Phase 3- Repeat phases one and two with left arm if indicated, Iso'-Flex® *firmly* under right foot.

Phase 4- Anaerobic sprints - Progress to anaerobic sprints after 25 repetitions at normal speed can be done comfortably (see pages 56-57).

4. Extensor Wrist Curls:
   A. Exercise Benefit: Forearm extensors.
   B. Starting Position: Sit in chair and place Iso'-Flex® *firmly* under your right foot. Hold handle in your right hand with palm down. With elbow bent, support forearm on thigh with wrist and hand extended just beyond right knee.

Extensor Wrist Curls

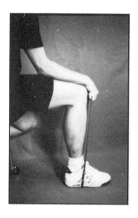

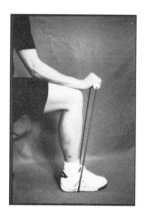

Starting Position

Exercise Action

   C. Exercise Action:
   Phase 1- From wrist-down (flexed position), slowly raise hand and bend wrist back as far as possible. Hold *firmly* for 2 seconds.
   Phase 2- Return slowly to starting position. Repeat 5 times. Progress slowly to 25 repetitions.
   Phase 3- Repeat phases one and two with left arm if indicated, Iso'-Flex® *firmly* under left foot.
   Phase 4- Anaerobic sprints - Progress to anaerobic sprints after 25 repetitions at normal speed can be done comfortably (see pages 56-57).

5. Ulnar Wrist Curls:
    A. Exercise Benefit: Ulnar wrist extensors, wrist abductors
    B. Starting Position: Sit in chair and place Iso'-Flex® firmly under your *right foot*. Hold handle in your *right hand* with palm down and wrist slightly extended. With elbow bent, support elbow and forearm on right thigh.

Iso'-Flex® Ulnar Wrist Curls

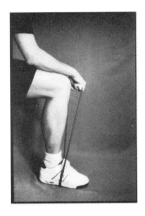

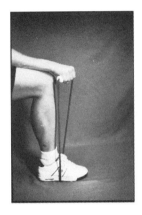

Starting Position

Exercise Action

C. Exercise Action:
    Phase 1- Slowly bend wrist sideways, bringing small finger side of hand as far to right as possible. Keep palm down at all times. Hold firmly for 2 seconds.
    Phase 2- Return slowly to starting position. Repeat 5 times. Progress slowly to 25 repetitions.
    Phase 3- Repeat phases one and two with *left arm* if indicated, Iso'-Flex firmly under *left foot.*
    Phase 4- Anaerobic sprints - Progress to anaerobic sprints after 25 repetitions at normal speed can be done comfortably (see pages 56-57).

6. Forearm Supination
   A. Exercise Benefit: Forearm supinators.
   B. Starting Position: Sit in chair and place Iso'-Flex® *firmly* under your *left foot.* Left foot should be positioned ten inches outside center of body. Hold handle in your *right hand* with palm down. With elbow bent, support elbow forearm on right thigh.

Iso'-Flex® Forearm Supination

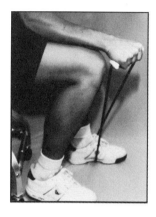

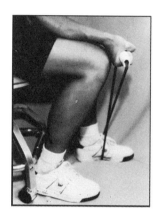

Starting Position   Exercise Action

   C. Exercise Action:.
   Phase 1- Slowly rotate forearm to palm up position. Hold firmly for 2 seconds.
   Phase 2- Return slowly to starting position. Repeat 5 times. Progress slowly to 25 repetitions.
   Phase 3- Repeat phases one and two with *left arm* if indicated, Iso'-Flex® *firmly* under *right foot.*
   Phase 4- Anaerobic sprints - Progress to anaerobic sprints after 25 repetitions can be done comfortably at normal speed (see pages 56-57).

III. Isometrics Plus Program

When the isotonic and Iso'-Flex® programs have progressed beyond one week, the isometrics plus program is started. These exercises should be done several times a day.

These exercises offer the additional opportunity to strengthen the finger, hand, and wrist muscles, many of which originate in the forearm.

Several times throughout the day, every day, repeat the exercises which follow. In the early stages of these exercises, do them with elbow bent at your side, forearm horizontal (parallel to ground). As you progress, straighten (extend) the elbow somewhat; do these exercises with the arm in front of you or at your side. The final goal of these exercises is to repeat each one with the arm extended (elbow straight but not locked). This position results in the maximum tension being placed on the muscles and tendons and is therefore the most effective. It is also the most demanding position and has the most potential for producing pain.

1. Finger Extension:
   A. Exercise Benefit: Strengthen wrist and finger extensor muscles.
   B. Starting Position: Place thick rubber band around thumb and fingers between the tip and middle knuckle joints in a position where the rubber band is stable. Start with the finger tips and thumb gently touching (eg. pinched position).

Isometric Plus Finger Extension

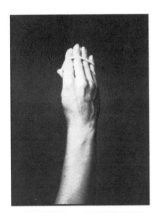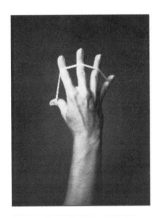

Isometric Relaxed Position   Isometric Plus Finger Extension

   C. Exercise Action:
      Phase 1- Actively pull fingers and thumb into fully straightened position, opening the hand wide. Hold for 1 second.

Phase 2- Slowly release hand and return to starting position.
Repeat until fatigue occurs (usually requires 25-30 repetitions).
Phase 3- Optional: Repeat phases one and two with opposite hand.
D. Speed: Moderate.

2. Hand Squeeze:
    A. Exercise Benefit: Strengthens wrist flexor and extensor muscles.
    B. Starting Position: Hold a tennis ball in hand.
    NOTE: You may need to start more easily with a nerf or racquet ball, and
    progress to a tennis ball, which is more demanding.

Isometrics Plus Hand Squeeze

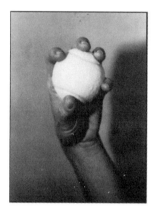 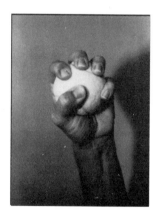

Relaxed Position   Squeeze Position

C. Exercise Action:
    Phase 1- Squeeze ball firmly and hold for 6 seconds.
    Phase 2- Slowly release ball. Repeat to fatigue.
    Phase 3- Optional: Repeat phases one and two with opposite hand.

Anaerobic Sprints (Iso'-Flex®)

Sport muscle activity occurs at high speed (often in milliseconds, e.g., 1/1000 second). As a final conditioning or rehabilitative exercise phase prior to work or sport activity return, it is recommended that high speed sprints be done (this also increases work endurance by working the muscle without an immediate oxygen supply, e.g., anaerobic exercise). It should be appreciated that most sports activities often occur in sudden bursts with temporary oxygen deficit to the muscle.

The technique of Iso'-Flex® sprints is to do each exercise in good form, but as rapidly as possible until the muscle fatigues.

CAUTION: This technique should *not* be used until the normal rehabilitative strength end points (isotonic and Iso'-Flex®) can be fully completed without discomfort for the specific exercise in question.

Anaerobic Sprint Technique

Start with 5 sprints of each exercise and gradually increase to 25 or more until muscle fatigue. Recommended exercises include flexor wrist curls, extensor wrist curls, pronation, and supination. If pain occurs with the sprints decrease repetitions or stop sprints and check with your physical therapist or doctor.

IV. Supplemental Resistance Exercises for Entire Arm and Trunk

The elbow exercises as noted on the prior pages are the key exercises for both lateral and medial tennis elbow. There are many circumstances when additional exercises are needed.

Tennis elbow is commonly (at least 50% of the time) associated with a "domino effect" of weakness and injury in the adjacent areas of the arm, shoulder, neck and upper trunk. Accurate examination of these areas is essential as the patient may be unaware of these deficiencies. When these deficits or injuries (such as shoulder rotator cuff tendinitis and or neck osteoarthritis) are present, it is strongly recommended that additional exercises be done. The supplemental exercises in association with tennis elbow most commonly prescribed at Virginia Sportsmedicine Institute are the following:

1. Biceps Curl (arm)
2. Triceps French Curl - Military Press (arm)
3. Virginia Sportsmedicine Institute, Inc. - rotator cuff basic foundation exercises (shoulder)

4. Virginia Sportsmedicine Institute, Inc. scapular - thoracic exercise program (mid-back)
5. Neck strengthening and flexibility programs
6. Shoulder flexibility program

The above areas for supplemental exercise are often critical to the tennis elbow program as deficiencies in these body parts will inevitably result in abusive overloading to the already sensitive and injured elbow tendons.

It has already been noted that other body areas should also be reviewed for abnormalities or strength deficits. These areas include the lower back and legs as even deficits in these more remote areas will affect the elbow (especially in the racquet sports which depend upon running and leg agility for proper technique).

V. Flexibility Exercises

Once you are well into your isotonic and Iso'-Flex® program while remaining relatively pain-free, begin *full* motion flexibility exercises. A full stretching program is delayed until now because it has been our experience that stretching prior to reasonable restoration of strength and healing often invites a recurrence of pain. CAUTION: Do these stretches only after you have completed a proper warm-up.

1. Forearm Stretch:
    A. Exercise Benefit: Full flexibility of wrist flexors and extensors
    B. Starting Position: Sit or stand holding arm comfortably in front of body, elbow completely straight, but not locked, palm up (supinated).

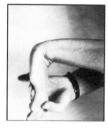 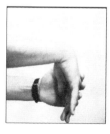 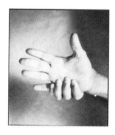

Forearm Flexibility
Supinated Position

Forearm Flexibility
Pronated Position

Forearm Flexibility
Rotations

C. Exercise Action:
Phase 1- Use opposite hand to slowly stretch the wrist back, fingers pointing toward floor. Hold for ten seconds and slowly release. Repeat 3 times.
Phase 2- With opposite hand, slowly stretch the wrist up into flexed position, fingers pointing toward ceiling. Hold for 10 seconds and relax. Repeat 3 times.
Phase 3- Starting position: Repeat phases 1 and 2 with palm down (pronated). Note: Fingers will be pointing opposite to supinated position.
Phase 4- Clasp hands, holding palms together, elbows straight but not locked. Slowly rotate hands over and back as far as possible three times. Firmly stretch at rotation end point. Hold for 3 seconds.
Phase 5- Repeat phases 1, 2 and 3 with other hand.

Rehabilitation for Highly Competitive Athletes

The programs discussed in this book for average sport participants (tennis, racquet ball, golf, squash, baseball, softball, etc.), occupational activities (word processing, meat cutting, assembly line activities, etc.), and performing arts (pianists, cellists, violinists, etc.) are those which have been developed while treating literally thousands of tennis elbow patients. They have proven effective in the usual circumstances and have stood the test of time.

The highly competitive sports and peforming arts athlete involved in tournament or professional activities such as tennis, other racquet sports, baseball pitching, javelin throwing and golf often requires even more sophisticated and demanding rehabilitation to allow a successful return to the world of extremely high level performance. These athletes often have companion problems such as bone spurs, loose fragments, arthritis, loose ligaments and nerve pinch. These problems must also be tended to in the course of treatment.

The basic rehabilitation programs are, however, the same for recreational and elite athletes, but with progression to higher levels of resistance and endurance for the elite groups using isokinetic machines (hydraulic resistance with pre-set speed control), as well as, more demanding and higher resistance isotonic and Iso'-Flex® programs. The levels of basic aerobic and anaerobic fitness must, by necessity, also be greater.

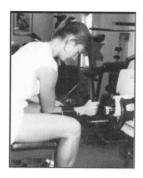

Cybex Isokinetic Exercise

Rehabilitation End Points

With the satisfactory completion of the rehabilitation program, a return to sports may be contemplated. The criteria which indicates that the program has been completed are as follows:

1. Ability to complete all rehabilitation exercise routines to full frequency and intensity with Phase 2 pain or less.
2. Pain free ADL's.
3. Objective testing that demonstrates normal balanced strength relationships between the forearm muscles of the injured vs. the non-injured side. For competitive athletes, a sophisticated isokinetic test such as Cybex is done. This type of testing is the most accurate and gives the most information concerning muscle balance ratios and muscle work capacity. For the lesser demands of the casual athlete, hand grip testing by dynamometer and circumferential measurement of forearm girth may suffice.

NOTE: The dominant arm is generally 10% stronger in grip strength than the non-dominant arm in the average person, and up to 25% stronger in the elite competitive racquet and throwing sport athletes.

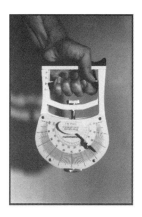

Dynamometer grip strength test

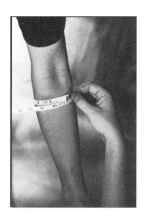

Circumferential forearm measurement. The dominant arm on average is 1/4 to 1/2 inch larger in average individuals and 3/4 to 1 inch larger in elite athletes.

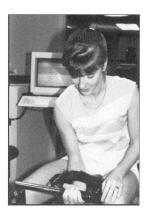

Cybex strength test

Transitional Exercise and Return to Sports

The goals of rehabilitation are to return injured or weakened tissue to normal. An average recovery from tennis elbow often takes 3 to 4 months. In addition, normal tissue is not necessarily ready for the rigors of competitive sport.

As such, once the rehabilitative process has been completed, transitional exercise is recommended. Chapter VIII discusses these issues in more detail. The principles are, however, as follows:

1. The end point of rehabilitation is best determined by objective testing (dynamometer grip or the more sophisticated Isokinetic testing/Cybex, for example).
2. Transitional exercise includes a graduated return to the specific sport or performance activity. It should be noted that performance activities have very different speeds, angles, ranges of motion, and use different muscle energy systems than rehabilitation exercise.
3. Other types of exercise including plyometrics (the ballistic use of bodyweight) can be helpful as transitional exercise.

4. It is prudent to obtain information from knowledgeable persons (coaches,trainers and medical personnel) concerning return to the specific sport or activity. Performance tests are often available for many specific activities.

Examples of Transitional Exercise

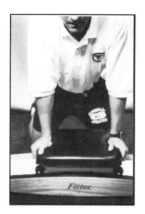 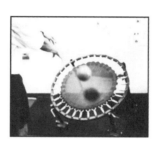 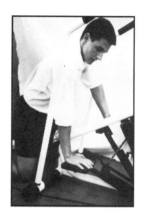

Maintenance Exercise

Once the rehabilitative process has achieved the goal of restoring the injured tissues to normal, the process is still not complete. Activities of daily living will not maintain fit tissue, and the rigors of sports or performance are often punishing and injury producing. Since sport and ADL's are not sufficient to maintain rehabilitated tissue, a maintenance program is a must. Otherwise retroversion to an unfit or re-injured status is likely.

The principles of maintenance exercise are as follows:
1. Maintenance exercise is indicated so long as the initial injury producing sport or activity is being continued.
2. Once fully returned to sport or performance activities, continue the full rehabilitation exercise program for 3 more weeks. If no pain is present, continue sports or performance activities and downgrade rehabilitation maintenance exercises to three times a week for 3 weeks, then two times week thereafter on a permanent basis.
3. Failure to do maintenance exercise invites re-injury.

Highlights of Chapter VI

1. The goals of rehabilitation are to encourage new blood supply, new healing cells, and new collagen protein to enter the injured tendon. Restoration of normal, pain-free strength, endurance and flexibility generally means these goals have been achieved.

2. Rehabilitation is a very precise undertaking. For best results, a series of properly staged resistance systems is recommended. These include:

   a. Isotonic weight resistance
   b. Iso'-Flex® tension cord resistance
   c. Isometric plus resistance
   d. Isokinetic resistance (usually in elite athletes)

3. Flexibility exercise is implemented after the resistance programs are well underway.

4. Many tennis elbow patients have companion deficiencies of the arm, shoulder, neck and upper back, and supplemental exercises must be done for these areas when deficiencies are present. Most patients are unaware that these defects are present. It is important, therefore, for the treating doctor to seek them out.

5. Transitional return to sport exercise and maintenance exercise are critical to prevent reinjury.

Chapter VII

Surgery

For most uncomplicated cases of tennis elbow, non-surgical rehabilitation can be expected to alleviate the injury. In those cases which don't respond to the conservative treatment and in the complicated case, surgery may become an option. In this circumstance specific considerations are appropriate.

Basic Reasons for Surgery:

1. Lack of response to a quality conservative treatment program.
   NOTE: Failure to respond to a *poor* conservative program or *lack of patient compliance* to an adequate program does not justify resorting to surgery. A proper effort with a good program (as presented in this book) should be instituted before failure is accepted.

The following clinical history or signs have often been noted to be present more often when failure of the conservative treatment occurs:

   a. The patient has received three or more cortisone injections.

   NOTE: We do not advocate cortisone injections as a primary treatment and do not use the criteria of failed cortisone injections as a reason for surgery. We do see, however, many patients referred from elsewhere, who have had multiple cortisone injections prior to our evaluation. It is possible that the selection of cortisone injection treatment reflects a more difficult case to begin with. In those cases in which the pain is so intense that it prevents the initiation of, or compliance with the rehabilitation program, a cortisone injection is appropriate. We strongly recommend, however, that every patient be fully aware of the reasons to use a cortisone injection before accepting this form of treatment. Cortisone by injection is anti-inflammatory (acting as a peripheral pain reliever) at the injection site. It *does not,* however, promote healing and tends to be detrimental in the long term by *weakening the tendon.*

The technique of injection, as well as, the kind of cortisone and number of injections are all important in determining the ultimate effect of the injection. The best injection site for lateral tennis elbow is usually in the triangular recess below the extensor brevis tendon. For medial tennis elbow, the best injection site is at the painful area and usually close to the tip of the medial epicondyle.

b.   Easy flow of injected fluids (e.g., novocaine type medication or cortisone).

NOTE: Our present recommended indication for cortisone injection is when other pain relief methods have failed and pain is so intense that compliance with the conservative treatment is compromised. This situation occurs approximately twenty percent of the time. The best technique for lateral tennis elbow injection is below the extensor brevis tendon. Easy flow of the cortisone indicates a significant tear or a major change (weakening) of the tissue in this region.

c.   Positive MRI test of elbow tendons. (This is a very new technology and findings are preliminary).

d.   Presence of calcium deposits on x-ray. This occurs approximately twenty-two percent of the time.

NOTE: Calcium does not cause the pain but does indicate an overall chronic problem.

e.   Mesenchymal syndrome: Presence of multiple tendinitis and nerve pinch symptoms in many body areas. Some patients have tendinitis in many areas at the same time such as both shoulders, tennis elbow in both elbows, or wrist nerve pinch (carpal tunnel syndrome). This occurs approximately fifteen percent of the time.

2.   Significant alteration of the quality of life.
Some patients find the intensity and chronic nature of their pain extremely compromising to their social, physical, emotional or economic well being. Under these circumstances surgery is an appropriate treatment choice.

If Surgery is Selected

Once surgery is selected as the proper treatment, other important factors must be considered for best success:

a. The surgical technique:
Surgical techniques have changed markedly in recent years. The older concepts of wrist, elbow and shoulder surgery were primarily designed for non-athletic and more elderly persons. Key changes in techniques have been made as recently as the time of this publication. Since medical care often improves, further advances are likely. The surgical techniques utilized at the Nirschl Orthopedic/Sportsmedicine Clinic have evolved over 1,000 surgical cases of tennis elbow. This surgical experience is one of the world's most extensive and has proven quite effective. Cure or major improvement of symptoms can be anticipated in 97% of lateral and medial tennis elbow surgical cases utilizing these techniques.

Posterior tennis elbow occurs more commonly with olecranon chondromalacia and loose fragments, and usually responds well in association with arthroscopic removal of fragments, but is somewhat less consistent in pain relief (especially for high demand athletes).

b. A quality supervised post-operative rehabilitation program:
The program in this book is well suited for the post-operative period. For full success, *the patient must do a credible job of rehabilitation.*

Some Technical Thoughts

As noted above, surgical techniques have been evolving dramatically in recent years. Our surgical experience has led to some concepts which should aid in the quest for maximum success. These newer concepts have been extremely helpful in improving the surgical success rate while decreasing the post-op rehabilitative time and effort. Discuss surgical concepts with your surgeon before any contemplated surgery and make sure he or she is a well qualified orthopedic surgeon with a good understanding of athletic injury and treatment concerning both the elbow and shoulder.

Elbow Surgery

1. The tendon pathology (injury) is usually located in the area of maximum tenderness to touch.

   These areas generally are:
   a. Lateral elbow - *Extensor Brevis tendon*
   b. Medial elbow - *Pronator Teres and Flexor Carpi Radialis tendons*
   c. Posterior elbow - *Triceps tendon*

It is usually best to remove and repair only those tissues involved in the injury. Older surgical techniques commonly called "tendon slides, releases, Bosworth procedure, etc." often release normal tissues and tend to result in poor or inconsistent pain relief, weakness or a prolonged rehabilitation time. The goal of surgery is removal of unhealthy, painful tissue, not release of tendon attachments.

NOTE: Although we use arthroscopic surgery widely for elbow arthritis and shoulder rotator cuff surgery, the elbow tendons cannot be reached easily with the arthroscope. Small open incisions are therefore best for elbow tendon surgery.

2. If Ulnar nerve pinch occurs at the medial elbow, ("funny bone nerve pinch") surgical decompression of the nerve pinch will help. In most instances, it is unnecessary to transfer the nerve forward.
   NOTE: In the past, forward (anterior) ulnar nerve transfer was thought to be necessary for operative success. Check this point closely with your doctor.

3. If calcium deposits occur, removal is appropriate, but under some circumstances not always necessary.

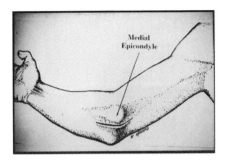

Surgical Incision

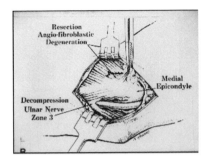

Resection Tendinosis -Decompression Ulnar Nerve

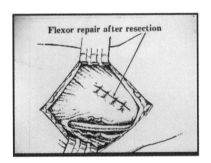

Repair of Tendons

Surgical Technique Medial Tennis Elbow and
Ulnar Nerve Pinch. Surgical technique
developed and commonly used at
Nirschl Orthopedic & Sportsmedicine Clinic

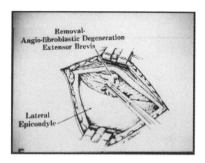

Surgical Excision of Tendinosis

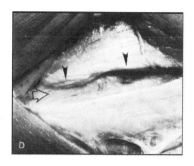

Surgical Photograph of Tendinosis (open arrow)

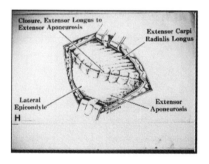

Repair of Tendons after Excision of Tendinosis

Surgical Technque Lateral Tennis Elbow
developed and commonly used at
Nirschl Orthopedic & Sportsmedicine Clinic

Final Surgical Thoughts:

The success of surgery is dependent upon many things. Certainly the surgeon must do his or her part, but the patient must be prepared to do his or her part as well. Positive mental attitude and the resolve to work hard in the rehabilitation effort are key factors to success. A specific post surgery rehabilitation plan is an additional key to success.

NOTE: *No* surgery can be guaranteed since uncontrollable factors can and do occur. With the above thoughts in mind, however, a high level of surgical success with return to sports or performance activity can be anticipated.

Highlights of Chapter VII

1. Although most patients respond to the conservative treatment program, surgical treatment, on occasion, is an appropriate option.

2. Surgical techniques have evolved, and the present techniques for lateral and medial tennis elbow as presented are highly successful. Posterior tennis elbow is less common as an isolated event, but is often associated with loose bone chips and combined arthroscopic surgery is often used successfully for posterior tennis elbow.

3. After-surgery rehabilitation programs of high quality are important to ensure maximum surgical success.

Chapter VIII

Transition Exercise: Return to Performance Activities

The completion of rehabilitation and restoration of fitness are major elements in the return to performance activity. It should be noted that performance activity often occurs at much faster speeds and much higher power ratios than either rehabilitation or fitness exercise. Therefore, a final step is needed to complete the successful transition back to performance activities. With these thoughts in mind, let us pursue the concepts of exercise including the goal of return to high performance.

General Concepts

There are 3 basic exercises:
1. Rehabilitation
   The goal of rehabilitation exercise is to restore injured, diseased or weakened tissue to normal.
2. Fitness
   The goal of fitness exercise is to take normal tissue and progress to better normal or super normal level.
3. Performance (sports, occupational or performing arts)
   The goal of this category of exercise is to win, produce a product, enhance a skill level or perform a task or service.
   NOTE: Since performance exercise activities occur at different exercise angles and speeds than rehabilitation exercises, a gradual return to performance activities is not only prudent but critical to prevent recurrent injury and to enhance performance.

In the transition back to full level performance the following is recommended:
1. Full completion of the rehabilitation program.
2. Return to normal strength, endurance, and flexibility as measured by dynamometer (Cybex or other).
3. Satisfactory completion of anaerobic sprints.

4. Use of protective techniques including:
   a. proper sports or occupational techniques
   b. Appropriate Count'R-Force® bracing
   c. gradual progression in duration and intensity of activity
5. Use of return practice schedules as outlined in this book or taught by knowledgable coaches and supervisors (see pages 75 - 78).
   NOTE: The practice schedules are meant to be guidelines. Rigid adherence to the schedule is not indicated in many cases as individual variations are common. The key point is gradual return.
6. Supplemental transition exercises, such as plyometrics, dynamic eccentric loading, agility and specific performance drills are recommended. This topic is broad in scope, and is addressed in detail in other publications.

Baseball

The major elbow tendon difficulty in baseball throwing is medial tennis elbow. It is important to note that other companion problems are common, especially in baseball pitchers. These maladies include:

1. Ulnar nerve pinch at the medial elbow,
2. Medial collateral ligament injury with elbow laxity (valgus),
3. Chondromalacia, arthritis and loose bone chips at back of the elbow (olecranon joint).

It is important to know if any of the above problems are present, as these problems will alter or compromise any return schedule for medial tennis elbow tendinosis.

Technique Considerations

Allowing the elbow to drag behind the body in baseball throwing is punishing to the medial elbow. To prevent elbow drag, the following concepts in the throwing techniques are suggested:

1. Avoid premature opening up of the pelvis,
2. Avoid dropping the arm below a $90°$ angle to the body at any time in the throwing motion,
3. Avoid extending the elbow beyond $90°$ when throwing curves and sliders,

4. Don't let the plant foot (left foot in right-handed pitcher) stray beyond the body midline, or extend the stride to far forward.
    NOTE: Check with a knowledgable coach concerning these aspects.

Return Schedule Concepts for Baseball:

1. Do warm-ups (see Chapters V and IX) before all practice sessions.
2. Be sure rehabilitation has been completed.
3. Use Count'R-Force® brace during play.
4. Fitness programs should be commensurate with anticipated sports activity.
5. Transitional exercises:

Week one
   a. Easy looping throws of increasing distance, 90-120 feet, on a daily basis.
   b. Exercise for 5 minutes to start - progress to 20 minutes once or twice a day over a period of one week.

Week two
   a. Return to mound.
   b. Undertake throws of more level trajectory at no greater than 50% of pre-injury velocity.
   c. Exercise routine for 5 minutes to start - progress to 15 minutes once or twice a day over a period of one week.
   d. No sliders or curve balls.

Week three
   a. Gradually increase velocity as comfort permits for fast balls. Remain at 50% velocity for curves.
   b. No sliders.

Week four
   a. Gradual return to normal pitching routine over the next 2 weeks, including fast balls, curves and sliders.

Tennis

Return to tennis is often a complex affair. The variety of medical problems (lateral, medial and posterior tennis elbow and nerve pinch) and stroke patterns (e.g., serve, overhead, ground strokes, volleys, lobs, spins and grip variations) often make the return quite challenging, especially in the elite athletic group.

As with baseball, a gradual return is recommended and careful review of stroke technique and equipment by a knowledgeable medical professional and coach is critical.

To prevent elbow tendon overuse, the following techniques are suggested:
1. Avoid late strokes.
2. Use your body weight and shoulder motion for power.
3. Avoid rigid jumbo sized racquets.
4. Keep string tension soft,
5. Use proper grip size,
6. Avoid exaggerated spin shots.

Return Schedule Concepts for Tennis:
1. Do warm-ups (see Chapter V and XI) before all practice sessions.
2. Be sure rehabilitation is completed.
3. Use Count'R-Force® brace at all times during play.
4. Do fitness programs on continuing basis.
5. Individual circumstances often are present and variation from the practice schedule guidelines on pages 77 and 78 may be appropriate.

Lateral Tennis Elbow Practice Schedule
Return Guidelines
Progress If No Pain Increase

Tournament Player

Day	Duration	Technique
1	15 min.	F only
2	20 min.	F; FL; few FV
3	30 min.	F; FL; FV; Few O (to F court only)
4	35 min.	F; FL; FV; O; Few S
5	40 min.	F; FL; FV; O; S (no SL,T, or AT)
6	45 min.	as day 5
7	1 hr.	as day 6
8	1 hr. a.m.	F; FL; FV; O; S (no SL or AT); few B (two handed)
9	1 hr.	F; FL; FV; O; S (no AT); B; (no BV)
10	1 hr. (a.m.)	F; FV; L; O; S; (no AT) B; (no U)
	15 min. (p.m.)	F; FL; O
11	1 hr. (a.m.)	as day 10
	20 min. (p.m.)	as day 10
12	1 hr. (a.m.)	as day 11
	30 min. (p.m.)	F; FV; L; O;
13	1 hr. (a.m.)	F; FV; L; O; S; B; few BV (no U)
	45 min. (p.m.)	F; FV; L; O; S
14	1 hr. (a.m.)	F; FV; L; O; S; B; BV
	1 hr. (p.m.)	as a.m.
15		Resume normal practice/play schedule

Recreational Player*

Day	Duration	Technique
1	15 min.	F only
2	30 min.	F; FL; few FV
3	35 min.	F; FL; FV; Few O
4	45 min.	F; FL; FV; O
5	1 hr.	F; FL; O; S; Few B (2 handed)
6	1 hr.	F; FV; FL; O; S; BV (2 handed); B
7	1 hr.	F; FV; L; O; S; B; BV (2 handed); B
8	1 hr.	F; FV; L; O; S; B
9		Resume normal practice/play schedule

*Progression for recreational player refers to actual playing days, not chronological days.

Code for Tennis Practice Schedules

F = Forehand	T = Topspin
FV = Forehand Volley	AT = American Twist
S = Serve	L = Lob
U = Underspin	BL = Backhand Lob
B = Backhand	FL = Forehand Lob
SL = Slice	O = Overhead
BV = Backhand Volley	

Caution

1. Use Lateral Count'R-Force® at all times.
2. Hit easily - hit through the ball.
3. Stay in balance.
4. Stay in hitting zone.
5. No late strokes.
6. Keep eye on ball.
7. Two-handed backhand is protective.
8. Ice sore areas immediately after play.

Medial Tennis Elbow Practice Schedule
Return Guidelines
Progress If No Pain Increase

Tournament Player

Day	Duration	Technique
1	15 min.	B only (2 handed); L (no late strokes)
2	20 min.	B (2 handed); L; Few F (2 handed)
3	30 min.	B; L; Few F (no T); F; (no late strokes), (no topspin)
4	35 min.	B; L; BV; F (no T)
5	40 min.	B; L; BV; F (no T); Few O (to F court only)
6	45 min.	B; L; BV; F (no T); O (to F court only)
7	1 hr.	as day 6
8	1 hr.	B: L; BV; F (no T); FV; (no late strokes ever!)
9	1 hr.	All strokes easy
10	1 hr. (a.m.) 15 min. (p.m.)	as day 9 B; L; F
11	1 hr. (a.m.) 30 min.	B; l; BV; F (no T); O; FV; S; (no T or AT) B; L; BV; F; (no T)
12	1hr. (a.m.) 45 min. (p.m.)	B; L; BV; F; O; FV; S; (no T or AT) B; L; BV; F; O
13	1 hr. (a.m.) 1 hr. (p.m.)	same as day 12 same as a.m.
14	1 hr. (a.m.) 1 hr. (p.m.)	B; L; BV; F as a.m.
15		Resume normal practice/play schedule

Recreational Player*

Day	Duration	Technique
1	15 min.	L only
2	20 min.	L; B
3	30 min.	as day 2
4	40 min.	L; B; F; BV
5	45 min.	L; B; F; BV; few O
6	1 hr.	L; B; F; BV; O
7	1 hr.	L; B; BV; F; O; few S
8	1 hr.	L; B; F; BV; O; S; F; (no late strokes ever!)
9		Resume normal practice/play schedule

*Progression for recreational player refers to actual playing days, not chronological days.

Code for Tennis Practice Schedules

F = Forehand	T = Topspin
FV = Forehand Volley	AT = American Twist
S = Serve	L = Lob
U = Underspin	BL = Backhand Lob
B = Backhand	FL = Forehand Lob
SL = Slice	O = Overhead
BV = Backhand Volley	

Caution

1. Use Medial Count'R-Force® at all times.
2. Hit easily - hit through the ball.
3. Stay in balance.
4. Stay in hitting zone.
5. No late strokes.
6. Keep eye on ball.
7. Avoid frame shots.
8. Ice sore areas immediately after play.

Highlights of Chapter VIII

1. Sports and performance activities are done at specific speeds, angles, range of motion and use muscle energy systems which are specific to the performance activity.

2. A transition program from rehabilitation to performance activities is therefore important to prevent injury and enhance performance.

Chapter IX

Warm-up Routines for Baseball, Tennis and Golf

In each sport, routines of warm-up can enhance enjoyment and performance while protecting from injury. The following routines for baseball, tennis and golf have proven successful in accomplishing these goals.

Baseball Pitching Warm-up (General Concepts):

To pitch a seven or nine inning game takes sensational body and arm stamina and strength. Proper total body strength, endurance, flexibility, aerobic, anaerobic and heat training should long precede any attempt at competitive pitching.

Each warm-up pitch may increase arm fatigue later in the game. Throw only enough hard pitches to groove your motion. The *major part* of the warm-up should not include actual hard pitching.

Check with your doctor and get his/her approval concerning the following routine.
Phases of Warm-up:
    Phase 1- If mildly stiff, take two buffered aspirin (with doctors approval) thirty minutes before the game.
    NOTE: Phases 2 and 4 should be included in your routine (especially for highly competitive events) if facilities and personnel permit, otherwise go on to Phases 3 and 5.
    Phase 2- One hour before game, heat shoulder and elbow with heating pad, hot shower, etc., for five minutes.
    Phase 3- Massage the shoulder and elbow for five minutes with mineral oil or a methyl salicylate product such as Craemergesic, Ben-Gay, etc. If a trainer is available, keep your arm elevated on two pillows and have him/her massage your arm from hand to shoulder.
    Phase 4- Fully relax and hang with both hands from a chinning bar for sixty seconds.

Phase 5- When on the field, jog or do jumping jacks until light sweat occurs.

Phase 6- Do the elbow flexibility exercises as noted on pages 58-59.

NOTE: Flexibility exercises can be done before Phase 4 if Phases 2 and 3 were completed.

Phase 7- Do your usual flexibility program for shoulder, back and legs.

Phase 8- Do your usual pre-game throwing, grooving and agility drills.

NOTE: Throw only enough to groove your motion. Do not cause fatigue.

Phase 9- Start easy throwing about one-half the usual distance and gradually lengthen throws to full distance.

Phase 10- When arm is loose, throw a few hard pitches to groove your final competitive motion.

Phase 11- Keep your warm-up jacket on at all times when not pitching in the game. If the day is cold and damp, consider wearing a thermal undershirt.

CAUTION: If undershirt becomes sweated, you may chill excessively. Change to a dry undershirt in a warm area (car or bus if necessary) between innings.

Baseball Pitching Cool-Down

The following cool-down program is designed for more highly competitive situations such as senior high school to professional play. Components of the program may be indicated in less competitive environments, but it is unlikely that the complete program will be appropriate.

1. Take two buffered aspirin (if your doctor approves) immediately after completing the activity.
2. Take a quick shower, keeping arm elevated. Dry thoroughly.
3. Lie down and elevate arm on two pillows.
4. Apply crushed ice in bags to medial elbow and shoulder.
   NOTE: Ice Strap™ is extremely helpful for convenience and effectiveness. If necessary, take ice to playing area in a thermos or cooler.
5. Squeeze racquet ball or nerf-type ball gently while elevating and icing the arm.
6. Ice arm for 15 to 30 minutes. If arm is badly swollen, ice and elevation may be indicated for two hours or more (30 minutes on and

skin redness).
7. If arm is badly swollen, an air compression device such as a Jobst Air Compression Sleeve, if available, will help eliminate the swelling.
8. When major swelling is gone (usually the next day) you may throw lightly only after proper warm-up. Return to pitching rotation when no further pain or swelling exists (usually four days for a professional pitcher).
NOTE: At the professional level general body muscle massage by an athletic trainer or other trained personnel has proved to be effective in relieving general muscle stiffness and soreness after competitive activity.

Tennis Warm-up

Tennis warm-up is similar to baseball in the early phases. Basic tennis motions are more protective than baseball. Tennis play is also more consistent than the intermittent inning driven activities of baseball pitching. In warm weather, therefore, it may be unnecessary to complete all the phases of tennis warm-up.

Phases of Warm-up (see pg. 73-74)
Phase 1- If mildly stiff, take two buffered aspirin (with doctor's approval) thirty minutes before each match.
Phase 2- If weather is cool, warm arm with infra-red lamp, heating pad, hot shower, etc., for five to ten minutes.
Phase 3- Massage shoulder and elbow for two minutes with a methyl salicylate product such as Craemergesic, Ben-Gay, etc.
Phase 4- Do jumping jacks or jog until light sweat occurs.
Phase 5- Do the elbow flexibility exercises as noted on pages 58-59.
Phase 6- Do your usual shoulder, back and leg flexibility exercises.
Phase 7- Do your usual pre-match tennis stroke grooving and agility drills.
NOTE: Hitting easy overheads first is more efficient in getting all body parts involved early. It is important that you include all stroke motions, including the serve and overhead in your warm-up.

Tennis Cool-down

If no injury symptoms are present, no specific cool-down is indicated. If shoulder, elbow or wrist symptoms are present, however, the program as outlined for baseball may be followed. In general, major swelling is unlikely to occur following tennis. Return to competitive tennis is often possible the same or following day. At the professional level, massage is often utilized effectively to relieve muscle stiffness and soreness between matches.

Golf Warm-up

Golf involves a variety of motions and muscle groups. Shoulder and back problems are commonplace. Medial tennis elbow is an important injury in the trailing arm as is lateral tennis elbow in the leading arm of the golf swing. In the nice heated environment of an outdoor, sun drenched golf course; warm-up is easily achieved. However, a major hazard occurs in cold weather. Under these circumstances, attention to full warm-up may be critical, yet is often overlooked (unfortunately inviting injury).

Check with your doctor and get his/her approval concerning the following routine.

Phases of Warm-up:
Phase 1- If mildly stiff, take two buffered aspirin (with doctor's approval) thirty minutes before tee off time.
Phase 2- Massage elbow vigorously with methyl salicylate product such as Craemergesic, Ben-Gay, etc. for 1-2 minutes.
Phase 3- Use proper clothing, including a jacket, throughout the golf round.
Phase 4- Do light jumping jacks, jogging, etc. to warm-up.
Phase 5- Do elbow flexibility exercises as noted on pages 58-59. Add neck, shoulder, back and leg stretches. A golf club can be a useful flexibility exercise tool.
Phase 6- Take a series of practice swings including woods and long irons.

Highlights of Chapter IX

1. Warm-up routines are important to prevent injury and enhance performance.

2. Body heat elevation to an end point of a light sweat is recommended.

3. Do not fatigue with sports motions prior to sports play.

EPILOGUE

The recreational boom is upon us. The benefits of athletic participation far outweigh the hazards, nonetheless, problems do occur. We believe, however, that the large majority of arm injuries can be resolved or prevented by the techniques outlined in this book. In fact, non-exercise is usually more hazardous to your health!

Overall, the principles and techniques we have detailed are applicable to the enhancement of performance, as well as injury prevention and treatment. These principles are also in large part appropriate for problems in other body parts (such as shoulder tendinitis, shin splints, runner's knee, achilles tendinosis and plantar fasciitis).

We hope the information in this book proves as beneficial to you as it has to the thousands of patients we have had the pleasure of serving over the years.

About The Authors

Robert P. Nirschl, M.D., M.S.

Dr. Nirschl is an actively practicing orthopedic surgeon in Arlington, Virginia. His contributions to the knowledge of orthopedic sportsmedicine are internationally recognized within the medical community. Active in competitive sports during school years, his interest in the orthopedic aspects of sportsmedicine was formulated after developing tennis elbow during orthopedic speciality training at the Mayo Clinic. Dr. Nirschl's initial research in the 1970's concerning the contribution of sports technique and equipment to sports injury resulted in many developments in sports injury treatment including concepts and techniques for the conservative and surgical care of tendon injuries to the elbow and shoulder. In 1974, Dr. Nirschl was one of the first physicians in the United States to incorporate the use of Nautilus type resistance machines in injury rehabilitation programs. This innovation resulted in the formation of Virginia Sportsmedicine Institute.

In 1987, the United States Tennis Association invited Dr. Nirschl, along with tennis champion, Stan Smith; sports psychologist, Jim Loehr; sports biomechanist, Jack Groppel; and orthopedic surgeon, Ben Kibler to initiate development of the USTA Player Development and Sports Science Programs. Dr. Nirschl is the founding director of sports medicine fellowship training programs in orthopedic and family practice in association with the Nirschl Orthopedic & Sportsmedicine Clinic and Arlington Hospital. He also holds the position of clinical associate professor of orthopedic surgery at Georgetown University. Dr. Nirschl served as medical consultant to the Presidents Council on Physical Fitness and Sports during the Reagan administration and currently serves on national committees for the American Orthopedic Society for Sportsmedicine, and the American Academy of Orthopedic Surgery. He acts as consultant and physician for professional, college and recreational athletes, including local Virginia high schools and Marymount University. Dr. Nirschl has lectured in England, Italy, France, Spain, Germany, Canada and Mexico, as well as, 39 of the states in the continental United States. He holds 4 U.S. patents and has contributed to and authored many orthopedic and sportsmedicine educational materials in numerous medical journals and books including video and audio formats. Dr. Nirschl enjoys tennis, skiing, jogging, walking and swimming with his wife, family and friends.

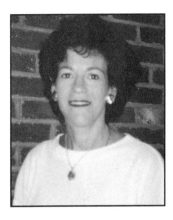

Janet Sobel, P.T.

Janet Sobel, P.T, has spent over 15 years specializing in the prevention and treatment of athletic injuries of the upper extremity. These programs and concepts are based on the foundation of scientific research combined with the clinical experience of work with professional and recreational athletes as clinical director of Virginia Sportsmedicine Institute. Ms. Sobel served as a member of the United States Tennis Association's Sport Science Committee and was the principal developer of the USTA's tennis flexibility program. She is currently a consultant to the Sport Science committee and to the Senior Fitness and Sports Foundation, an organization devoted to research and information dissemination on fitness and injury prevention among seniors. Ms. Sobel is on the editorial board of Rebound, a physician-patient communication publication developed by the Athletic Counseling and Treatment Institute. She has lectured and written extensively in the areas of sports injury prevention and rehabilitation.

Ms. Sobel is currently the Clinical Coordinator of Suburban Physical Medicine Center at Chevy Chase, Maryland.

Medical Sports, Incorporated Publications and Products

Iso'-Flex® Exercise
Count'R-Force® Braces

Lateral Elbow Brace	- for lateral tennis elbow
Medial Elbow Brace	- for medial tennis elbow
Radial Carpal Wrist Brace	- for carpal tunnel
Radial Ulnar Wrist Brace	- for ulnar side wrist
Arch Brace	- for plantar fasciitis
Sports Corset	- for back support in performance
Patellar Stabilizer	- for patellar problems (runner's knee)
Shin Splint Brace	-for shin splints

For Current Pricing or Information Please Contact:

Medical Sports, Inc.
P.O. Box 7187
Arlington, VA 22207
Phone: (703) 525-8600